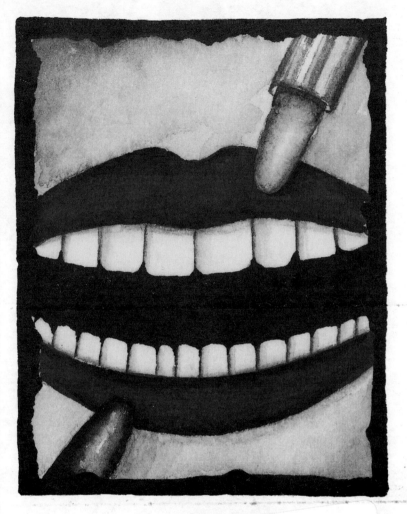

dear annie

dear annie

a no-nonsense guide to getting dressed

Annalisa Barbieri

illustrations by Clare Mackie

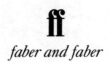

faber and faber

First published in 1998
by Faber and Faber Limited
3 Queen Square London WC1N 3AU

Typeset by Faber and Faber Ltd
Printed in England by Clays Ltd, St Ives plc

dear annie is a registered trademark

A CIP record for this book
is available from the British Library

ISBN 0-571-19628-4

2 4 6 8 10 9 7 5 3 1

this book is dedicated to
Luisa & Quinto
with all my love

contents

the directories

acknowledgements

Since the first 'Dear Annie' appeared in the *Independent on Sunday* in 1995, several people have nurtured the column. But even before its debut, there were those who gave me guidance and those I assisted; and with each of them I gathered a little bit more knowledge and learned a little bit more about fashion. It is therefore very important that those in the chain of events bringing me to this book are thanked:

Winston G. Dixon, my very first boss at the Home Office, who taught me nothing about fashion (other than that he liked see-through socks), but lots about office politics. Beverley Cable, for giving me that first foot in the fashion door, over a decade ago now. Simon Kelner, my first ever editor (at the *Observer*), who gave me my own page to nurture. Iain R. Webb, who taught me how to become even more efficient and organized when I worked with him at *The Times*. Lowri Turner for giving me so many articles to write when she was at the *Evening Standard*. Richard Askwith, perhaps the best copy-editor in the Western world and then editor of the 'Sunday Review', for asking me to come to the *Independent on Sunday* in the first place. To Liz Jobey, whom I worked with for only a few months but whose expert journalistic guidance I shall not forget. Jo Dale, for suggesting me to Sue Matthias, my editor on 'Real Life' for over two years, whom I'd also like to thank, hugely, for the chances she has given me and for letting me get on with it. Becky Gardiner, who nurtured and encouraged me in the early days. Clare Mackie, for always being a delight to deal with and for her sublime illustrations. To my colleagues Laura, Linda and Louisa for understanding Annie's made-up words and not trying to change them. Thank you to Jan Dalley and Suzi Feay for their book guidance; and to Peter Wilby and Rosie Boycott for all their support. A really big thank you to Jenny Turner for raving about me at dinner with a certain man called Giulio. To dearest Zoe Brown, who has had to put up with ceaseless banter and chatter and then stony book-writing silence, never once getting offended – and for helping to update the 'men and boys' chapter, her specialist subject. To Imogen Fox, without whom there *would* have been a 'Dear Annie' book, but not this year. And lastly but still most importantly, thank you to my beloved Pete for lots of things but especially for making me a constant supply of fishie & mash.

introduction

I'm not exactly sure when I first thought of doing a fashion problem column called 'Dear Annie'. I used to read the excellent 'Cher Albert' column in the *Evening Standard*'s *ES* magazine, when Albert Roux would answer cooking problems in his charming, quirky way. Sometimes he would be extraordinarily helpful and at other times (a particularly memorable occasion was when some fellow asked his opinion of the microwave) he would be – gently – dismissive. But he was always very readable.

There was no fashion equivalent to Roux's fabulous little column. A couple of glossy magazines had questions and answers, but the questions were obviously made up to fit in with some recently launched product or shop opening and the answer to everything seemed to be to go to Manolo Blahnik's and buy a nice pair of shoes. The fact that not everyone could afford a pair of Blahnik's wonderful shoes, or lived near his shop in London, didn't seem to matter. These shallow columns were token 'help the people' questions and in reality were anything but. They were, I felt, aimed more at the industry than at the reader, and that laziness annoyed me.

What I wanted to do was write a column like (I fancied) they had in the forties and fifties, a column with a gentle authority that would answer genuine questions (and yes, all the letters in 'Dear Annie' are genuine) from real people, all over the UK (and the world on some occasions). And wherever possible, the answer would be tailored to their budget and where they lived. 'Dear Annie' is not a lazy column, because real problems are difficult. Real people can't all wear the latest Gucci trousers: they may be too short or too tall, too fat or too broke; they may not live anywhere near a Gucci shop. I knew it wouldn't be easy or particularly glamorous, but I never dreamed it would be so much bloody fun either.

When the 'Real Life' section of the *Independent on Sunday* was first being talked about, back in the spring of 1995, it seemed to be the ideal place to have such a column. Sue Matthias, then editor of 'Real Life', went for the idea immediately and on 13 August 1995 'Dear Annie' appeared for the first time. The questions answered then were all genuine but from friends and colleagues. There was no way for the general public to know about it, yet. For the next few weeks the problems continued to be provided by people I knew; at one point, I wondered if indeed there would ever be any 'real' questions. Maybe people didn't need 'Annie'. (The name comes from the one person in the world who is allowed to call me Annie, a family friend called Pam, whose catchphrase when I was a teenager was 'Oh, *no*, Annie!')

But slowly the letters started to trickle in, and today the 'Dear Annie' column receives about 150 letters and e-mails a week. (When the column got an e-mail address in early 1997, the amount of men who wrote in shot up so that now there is about an even mix.) Letters from young ladies asking how to wear the latest skirt length, old ladies writing in about their slippers, teenagers asking about skatewear and what to do about their mum's old coat, men wondering where to buy *their* wedding outfits, and lots and lots of letters about bras. The youngest readers to write in have been eight years old, the oldest about ninety and the cross-section is huge. Some letters are funny, some – from post-mastectomy women especially – very sad, but all are lovely to read. Over the three years that Annie has now been going, regular correspondence has built up with some readers: David of London, Barbara of Hants, the Reverend Richard Curtis, Keith Lysons, JL from California. Despite the 'personal correspondence will not be entered into' rider at the end of the column, I quite often do.

Writing under a pseudonym of sorts is incredibly liberating. Once the research is done, 'Dear Annie' is ludicrously easy to write because it is the real me. And yet, bizarrely, Annie has a life of her own. The moment I sit down, each week, to write the column, I get into character; indeed, I think of Annie as another person altogether, which is why I often refer to her in the third person. I wanted people to understand early on that Annie wasn't perfectly shaped (I'm not), so they wouldn't feel intimidated about writing in to her. But this was difficult to get across in print. So one day I decided that Annie would have children. Four of them. A mother of four children would understand other people's problems; she too would have lumps and bumps to hide. Naturally, being a good Catholic, I had to give Annie a husband. I was tempted, at first, to make him something exciting and poetic but decided this was cheating, so Mr Annie became a pig farmer. (Coincidentally, the wonderful illustrations for the column are done by Clare Mackie, whose father *was* a pig farmer so for a while she would send me *Pig Farmer's Weekly*, so I could stay *au courant* of the piggie world.) There was to be little glamour in the Annie household.

As the letters poured in, it became obvious that there were certain problems that affected lots of people. The first was that people with bigger than average-sized feet found it really difficult to find shoes that fitted properly, let alone that were fashionable. So, in the column on Sunday, I asked for people to write in if they had 'big' feet and knew of any useful contacts, and I also asked for shops and manufacturers to get in touch if they made shoes in sizes bigger than the norm. Most other problem pages provide leaflets covering oft-asked questions ('Send in for my fact sheet on impotence'), so I thought it would be a good idea if Annie also had these. Thus the first directory was born – a nationwide list of useful contacts called the 'Big Shoe' directory. Others followed: 'Size 16 Plus', 'Dress-makers', etc. They are a phenomenal success and we get hundreds of requests a week for copies – these are often sent out late at night when my saner colleagues have gone home. Updated and revised, all the directories appear at the back of the book.

When I first asked people to send in an SAE (the only payment required) for the 'Big Shoe' directory, I had vastly underestimated the response and was inundated. With a full-time job on the paper to attend to as well, I fell badly behind. Disapproving 'You've let us down, Annie' letters started to arrive and I felt guilty. This is when I decided it was time Annie had a fifth child. I needed a breathing space and surely no one would scold a pregnant woman.

They didn't. By now, the column had created a little world of its own. At times I would be nervous of not knowing the answer to a question, and often the illustrations for the column would be commissioned *before* I knew if I could even answer the question. But this also proved useful, because it showed that Annie was, ahem, human. It also gave readers the chance to write in and help –

something they do most generously with 'I know, I know!' letters that put me, and the original correspondent, out of our misery. The best and most touching example of this was when Dr Scott Samuel (see the 'Men and Boys' chapter) asked for help in finding a pair of old-fashioned black plimsoles in a size 11 or 12. When another reader wrote in saying that you could get them in Zimbabwe for a few pounds, I jokingly said that if anyone went, could they get Dr Scott Samuel a pair. And someone did; they went to Zimbabwe and remembered his size and everything.

Although Annie has transcended trendiness to become a cult, I don't think it is madly popular among certain élitist parts of the fashion industry, and this pleases me greatly because it means I have succeeded. Aaah, the fashion industry, a place I have frequented for eleven years. My initial foray into fashion was at the age of seventeen, when I went to my first ever fashion show – Norman Hartnell's, in his west London showroom. I sat surrounded by very old ladies who talked of their chauffeurs (the show finished early and some were momentarily left stranded in the gilt showroom). So I pretended I had a chauffeur too, even being brash enough to offer one old dear a lift home in 'my' car. She declined and I went home on a number 7 bus, winging it on a half-fare too, if I remember rightly. I was to return to Norman Hartnell some months later as an apprentice seamstress, a role I was fired from exactly one month later, for 'applying nail varnish and polishing my boots over the Queen Mother's [she was a client] chiffon'. But I had stayed long enough almost to fulfil a teenage ambition to 'make the Queen's clothes' – I did the pleating on and hemmed the dress the Queen Mother wore for Prince Harry's christening.

Four years later I went back into fashion, spending the next four and a half years as a PR, having to deal with the often brattish whims of fashion editors (which is enough to make anyone resolve never to be one). After this, I crossed to the 'other side' when I went to be fashion assistant at the *Observer*. But after fifteen months of intense calling clothes in for shoots, sending them all back again, booking models and going to all the shows, where I would try desperately to draw the outfits I saw on the catwalk (later I would never be able to tell if my scribblings were A-line skirts with a front split or wide-legged trousers), I left to become a freelance journalist who also wrote on Other Subjects.

I never felt pure fashion was for me anyway. I hate shopping. I know what it's like to go into a shop and see something you think will look fabulous, only to have your mental image smashed in the cruel reflective world of the changing room. I too can find shopping for clothes traumatic at times; I need therapy after some shopping experiences. And I fit within the 'normal' size ranges available in shops, so I can only *imagine* what it must be like for someone who doesn't.

This is what makes me most cross about the fashion industry: the way people who are older or bigger than the 'norm' are mostly ignored. And I know how they feel because I read their letters. Most women in this country are a size 16 and over; in four years' time 33 per cent of the UK population will be over fifty. No wonder, then, that when fashion pages cover these 'unpopular' subjects they are pounced upon with glee and people write in saying, 'Thank you, at last!' There should always, *always* be room for fashion shoots that are inspirational and aspirational, but they should be mixed with reality, and sometimes reality has a big bottom.

Still, to defend fashion journalists for a moment, let me explain that it isn't as easy as people think to do more realistic fashion. Clothes used for fashion shoots are invariably available only in a size 10 or 12; even the outsize ranges are available only in a size 16 for photographic purposes. When we've done size 16 fashion at the *Independent on Sunday* (or, heaven forbid, size 16 on a fifty-plus woman), we've had enormous trouble getting clothes from designers and PRs. Only threatened exposure in a national newspaper for non-cooperation forces them to comply and send us in the blasted clothes. And this *from manufacturers of clothes that are sold in a size 16 or over*. Sometimes the PRs say, *sotto voce*, that their clients 'know it's their main customers but they don't want to be obviously associated with them in a dedicated size 16 shoot'. You see, the money of a woman with a normal-sized bottom may be good enough, but it's just not glamorous. I sometimes think these ridiculous little people don't like older, fatter women because it makes them *afraid* of what they might one day turn into themselves.

The people I really blame for this are the retailers, the manufacturers and the designers, for they are just plain lazy. Because our Western 'ideal' is tall and fairly slim, it's easy to make something look good on a tall and ridiculously thin model. What's so hard is dressing clever: knowing how to do a tuck here, a pleat there, and being able to carry the whole thing off with *confidence*. Confidence! How is anyone above a size 14 meant to have confidence when they are ignored and so rarely catered for? When almost every model you see looks like she could do with a good sandwich? When you go into a shop and there are rails upon rails of size 8s and 10s and 12s (you would have thought that by now someone, somewhere would have worked out that sizes 14 and 16 are more popular and therefore ordered more of them) but nothing bigger?

Luckily, things are changing. With the advent of a more efficient Internet, customers will be able and more willing to communicate their wishes direct to the retailers (electronic communication is so much easier and quicker than asking to see the manager or writing a letter). People are getting more and more pleasure from their homes and their kitchens (just look at the influx of interior and foodie magazines in recent years) and not just their clothes.

Annie doesn't care what size people are; all she cares about is that everyone – be they skinny (yes, they have just as much right to exist, too), plump, trendy or not – has the *choice*, the best choice, to wear what they want. She thinks people shouldn't worry too much about clothes. And her greatest weapon is that she doesn't give a hoot about the industry, she doesn't care what's in, she doesn't pander to a particular designer just because he's advertised in the newspaper, she rarely goes to shows and if she does she doesn't care if she's seated in the front row or not.

This book, then, is a compilation of letters printed in the column over the past few years. The very topical questions, about the latest fashions, etc., couldn't be included, because they wouldn't be relevant by the time this book came out and that would just be frustrating for the reader. All the information printed – every phone number, address, name, colour and style – has been checked, updated and revised, but even so it can only be correct at the time of going to press. The best way to use the book is to read it and then, if you want specific information, go to the fabulous index, because the chapters are rather quirky. Incidentally, for those not familiar with the column, 'Johnny Loulou' means John Lewis (even some of its staff now refer to this magnificent department store as Johnny Loulou now).

Finally, I have for the last year had the great good fortune of having Imogen Fox working with me. Prior to this I had been very fussy indeed about who did the 'Dear Annie' research, and because I thought no one could ever be as fact-obsessed as I was, I found it easier to do it myself (standards, like good manners, are so important). Naturally, Miss Fox also worked on this book with me, endlessly researching, checking numbers, sizes and colours, stapling and restapling, copying and cross-referencing. Aside from my own, this book could not have been in better hands, so in a way *Dear Annie: A No-nonsense Guide to Getting Dressed* is also Imogen's book.

Annalisa Barbieri

dear annie

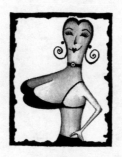

breasts
and how best to present them,
plus other useful information for the female form
*bras, corsets, girdles and tricks to stop
your bra strap showing*

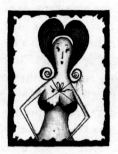

I bought ever such a sweet dress the other day from Top Shop. It has a high neck and cut-away arms. But I just cannot find a bra with straps that don't show and I don't want to go without. – *Barbara Evans, Abergavenny*

How wise of you not to leave your bosoms to gravity. You could wear a sports bra – the ones with racing backs would be perfect, as the front straps are also set in more than on conventional bras. But if you want to wear something prettier, or if you don't want to disrobe to reveal a rather unsexy sporting model, then wear your favourite, sexiest, blackest bra or body and tie a thin piece of elastic or ribbon to pull together (but not join) the two front (yes, front not back) straps. You'll have to experiment to see exactly what length of elastic/ribbon is best for you. This is good for two reasons: first, if a bit of bra does show, it's better that it's of the coronary-inducing variety. And, second, tying elastic/ribbon in this way pushes your quarter-pounders together to give you a cor-blimey silhouette. Elastic works best as it provides 'give' as you move (discreetly retire to the bathroom and cut it off before you undress), but if you plan to disrobe – or be disrobed – fast, then ribbon is recommended.

I followed your advice on how to wear a bra under a cut-out-arm dress and it worked brilliantly. I have a different problem: I have a great black Tactel short slip dress with shoestring straps from Marks & Spencer but I have to wear a bra (I'm a 36c). This means I can never wear it without something over the top. I think strapless bras look terrible on me – they give me a sausage-type chest – and I cannot afford to go to a fancy lingerie shop and have a bra made for me. Can I ever wear this dress and reveal my shoulders? – *Desperate, Dulwich*

Yes, it's great having bosoms but don't you wish you could get rid of them when you want to wear slip dresses with spaghetti straps? Don't you get sick of having to wear cute little T-shirts under the dress to hide the bra straps, or being forced to wear a bloody cardie? This trick takes only a little bit of time, but it works and can hopefully be used with a bra you already have. What you do is sew together the back straps of the dress, just for about an inch so that they come together at about the middle of your shoulder blades. This will make the neckline a bit higher, but will not make any difference to the dress you have. Then basically you do the same to the bra. Lengthen the straps so that they're so long that the metal 'buckle' bit is hidden by the dress at the back. Then sew it together at the back so that it matches up to the dress. You need a bra with simple flat straps (none of those fancy ruched numbers for this) and you can sew it and then slip it over your head (the same goes for the dress). It lifts your breasts up a treat and from the back it looks like you have on a multi-strapped dress. When you're done, you just unpick the stitches. Like my other bra trick, you can't undress in a hurry or when drunk, but who cares?

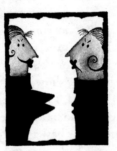

I have an older sister who is a completely different shape to me, she is flat-chested and I have a large bust. We still live at home and argue endlessly about sharing clothes. She won't let me near any of hers, saying I misshape them. The latest row was over her polo-neck jumper – she says it doesn't suit me as it makes my bust look bigger. I hate my bust anyway, but do you think she is right? – *Depressed, Middlesex*

It depends. A *baggy* polo-neck jumper – like any baggy jumper – is not the most flattering thing to wear if you have a large bust, as it falls from your chest to make you look bigger than you are. But a tight jumper with a well-fitting bra (go for something like Playtex's Cross Your Heart bra for torpedo-shaped breasts) will look fantastic. Let your sister have her moment of glory; there has been so much press of late on how attractive big bosoms are, she may well be feeling jealous. V-neck jumpers are anyhow far more flattering to a larger bust, so leave her with hers and hunt out one of your own.

**You seem very good on bra-related questions. I have a size 34D bust and want to wear a Wonderbra, but they only go up to a cup size C. Just because I have a D-cup bosom doesn't mean I don't also want to wear a Wonderbra.
– D. Collins, Derby**

Being a bit greedy, aren't you? Only joking. Well, the good news is that Wonderbra *do* go up to a D-cup. Or you may want to follow the advice of the American writer (and bosom and flirt expert) Dianne Brill and get a cup size smaller and a chest size bigger than you would normally wear (i.e., in your case a 36C). Hasn't done her any harm. Bravissimo (phone 07000 2442727 for a catalogue) have an equivalent to the Wonderbra which is the Cariche (CA01) and costs £25, in sizes 30–44, cup sizes D–G (but this is a bit misleading since the largest G cup is in a 34 back size). And the wonderful Margaret Ann (01985 840520) could order one from the mega-sexy Goddess range from America, so call her on 01985 840520. And yes, if I had £1 for every question I was asked about bosoms, I'd be really rich, so if anyone has a bra-related problem, please send £1 in with your query.

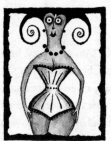

Where can I buy a corset for that 'nipped-in waist' look that is fashionable at present? The only ones I have seen are either silly prices or advertised by dubious 'specialist' shops. – Katie Wilson (Miss), Leicester

OK, Vollers The Corset Company in Portsmouth make very traditional corsets (all their patterns are 100 years old) which cost between £75 and £220, from sizes 18" (sharp intake of breath) to 40" (aaaaah), and there is a made-to-measure service. Call them on 01705 799030. They also do a catalogue. Rigby and Peller (0171 589 9293) do bespoke corsets from £500. Bellers of Islington, 193 Upper Street London N1 1RQ, tel: 0171 226 2322, do a full range of corsetry. The more old-fashioned laced-back stuff is available in sizes 26" to 44" waist, and the more modern stuff, which was described as 'Pride and Prejudice', comes in sizes 10–18, all from about £50. Margaret Ann (01985 840520) can offer all sorts of boned stuff, including an own-label range, from £80.

I have always had very bad posture and as I am getting older the problem is getting worse. (To the extent that if I don't find a solution soon, I will be staring my navel in the eye!) A friend once told me about 'posture bras'. Have you heard of such a thing? Can you suggest any other solution?
– Liela Hekmatyar, York

Yes, I have. A posture back bra does up at the front and has a full back, usually with criss-cross panels. It helps correct posture by supporting the upper back and encouraging you to keep your shoulders straight. Exquisite Form do two styles in their Fully range. The first is style no. 531: it comes in white, costs £16.99 and is available in sizes 34–44B/34–46/C 34–46D and 36–46DD. The second is style no. 565 and all details are the same except it costs £14.99. There is a freephone consumer advice line (0800 592553) which will put you in touch with stockists. It is also worth working on your latissimus dorsi (the muscles under the shoulders), as this will help take the strain of a larger bust (if that is your problem) and aid posture.

I have bought my girlfriend a slinky, strappy, backless dress. She is large-breasted, so must wear a bra, but all the ones she has show. I seem to remember that you've already given advice about this problem in your column – could you send me copies of your answers. – *Derek O'Carroll, Glasgow*

The advice I have given before was for wearing a bra with a dress with cut-out shoulders, or a strappy dress with a not-so-low back. With a backless *and* strappy dress, things are a little more difficult. Really, I do think you could have given a little more thought to your girlfriend's natural shape when making this otherwise generous offer. There is little alternative than for her to wear a basque with a very low back. Rigby and Peller in London (0171 589 9293) do some fabulous ones from about £40, but I know this is of little use to you in Glasgow. It is essential that the basque is well fitting, otherwise she may as well go without. I think the best bet for you is to ring Berlei (01525 850088), who do a brilliant range called Answers (like strapless bras, etc.), and from this they have a basque in sizes 32–38 and cup sizes A–D, costing £33, in black, white and pearl.

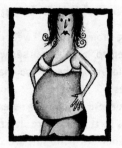

Who does a black nursing bra? My baby is due at the end of January and I always wear black underwear. Why are there only white ones?
– Yolanda, Peterborough

Just what is it with black underwear? Why isn't there more of it (everyday stuff as well as in regards to this question)? It isn't more expensive and yet it is regarded by retailers as somehow luxurious and we never, have the choice in black undies that we do in white. (I know the answer, of course: 'There just isn't as much call for it,' the manufacturers would say. Rubbish.) When I had my first child, Leonardo, there were no black nursing bras to be had at all, and I found that upsetting because I like my black underwear and after childbirth it is important to feel sexy, for oneself of course, even in small ways. Luckily things have changed. A bit. Blooming Marvellous (0181 391 4822) do one, style no. 1604 in sizes 34–40 and cup sizes B–DD: it's 95 per cent cotton/5 per cent elastane and costs £18.99. A brand called Emma Jane (enquiries 0181 599 3004) also makes a black nursing bra. Style no. 428 comes in sizes 34–40 and cup sizes B–E, costing £19. They also do a night nursing bra in black, style no. 371. This is to give your breasts support while you sleep; it can also hold breast pads in place (in case your breasts are weeping), costs £12.50 and comes in sizes M, L, XL and XXL. If you can't get to a store that sells them, they do send out the bras, though they are not mail order. The Active Birth Centre, 25 Bickerton Road, London N19 5JT, tel: 0171 561 9006, sells a great bra – the Bravado. It is a maternity and feeding bra made with Spandex and cotton, there are no back fastenings and it is pull-on (which isn't to everyone's taste as it's not as easy to get in or out of as more conventional do-up bras). It comes in black, white and a bold floral print, sizes 32B –46G, and it costs £22.95. They have a shop at the above address and also sell them mail order (0171 272 0987). This bra is also available from Bust Stop (0181 943 9733).

I think there is something wrong with me. I wear cleavage bras but some-how my breasts don't seem to 'meet', if you see what I mean. It's almost like the cups should be closer together. Do you have any ideas?
– Michaela Walker, St Ives

First, with bras such as these you have to wear them slightly differ-ently. Adjust the straps so that they are shorter than you would normally wear them. Then stuff the sides (i.e., like where the outside of your breast is, and underneath so you prop them up and in) with something like old tights. This doesn't sound very attractive but if you cut up a pair of old tights (preferably in the same colour as your bra) these are ideal for 'stuffing' as the fabric is pliable. Some bras also come with foam fillers, which are useful but never big enough. Make sure whatever you stuff your bra with isn't too 'solid' (which is why tights are so good) because not only is this uncomfortable but it will also give you a lumpy silhouette, and we don't want that.

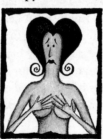

Can you advise me on how to dress to disguise the fact that my breasts are different sizes? Underwear isn't a problem as I wear a soft bra (I'm very small anyway), so it doesn't matter that one side is slightly too big. With a leotard I wear something loose on top, and when I go swimming I grit my teeth and scuttle between changing room and pool as fast as possible. Ordinary clothes are the problem. I can never wear anything that fits; I live in very loose things. I've heard that patterned fabric is best for this kind of thing, but I tried something on in a shop this morning with narrow horizon-tal stripes and it just seemed to accentuate the difference in size, and really upset me – I looked horrible. I don't know how obvious it is to other people but to me it's the most noticeable thing about me. Can you give me any tips? *– Jane Gibson, West Yorkshire*

I guess you're hoping that I can provide some miracle solution. I can't. I do so understand what it is like to try something on and feel that you look awful. This is why I rarely buy clothes – I can't bear to try them on in shops as my mood for the rest of the day is reliant on what I'll look like. The mistake you made, I think, is that stripes most probably will make things worse. Stripes can act like a grid system, accentuating all the wrong bits; by which I mean the bits *you* don't like. How different in size could your breasts be? Not much. The problem is in your head, and while I realize that this still makes it a problem (hence when we feel fat and ugly no matter what people say to make us feel better, we still feel fat and ugly), it is a problem that cannot be helped by any tips I can give you. Yes, patterned (abstract, floral, etc.) fabrics do 'fuzz' silhouettes and take the focus away from your shape and on to the pattern. You could also, I guess, pad one cup out slightly to make it look like the bigger breast. But there is *no reason at all* to skulk around wearing loose tops or to jettison yourself from changing room to swimming pool. The only thing that will effectively disguise your shape is to carry on wearing loose clothes, but do you really want to do this? What a waste. Unless you are a freak, in which case I would already have read about you in the *Sunday Sport*, any difference in the size of your breasts will be imperceptible. It is completely natural for one bosom to be slightly bigger than the other, usually the side that is more well developed (i.e., if you are right-handed the right-hand side of your body will usually be slightly larger). I am sorry if you were hoping for names and addresses of companies that do clothes to disguise this problem but I cannot advise you to hide something that is completely natural.

I bought the Marks & Spencer black Tactel slip that you've mentioned a few times. It is wonderful. However, as you know, it has shoestring straps and I cannot wear it without a bra. I've tried strapless ones, etc., but my bust is quite large (34DD) and believe me it does not look good with a strapless bra. It looks great with a bra underneath but obviously you can see it (the straps don't match up, one comes in more than the other). I thought if anyone could help, you could. Please do! – *Georgia, Plymouth*
OK, you have come to the right place. Thank you for your drawing to show me what the problem is, but it is easily solved. I know exactly what you mean. First, you have to get a black bra whose

strap is as simple as possible – no fancy lace, scalloping or beefy belt-size straps. Then put on the bra, put the dress on top and move the dress around by pulling it slightly under the arms (effectively stretching it out a bit) until the straps are one on top of the other, then just run a few stitches along (sort of under the arm) to join the dress to the bra. Tactel is a wonder fibre, although it is just good old nylon, which is the generic name for Tactel [for anyone wanting to swot up some more on fibres, read the 'Encyclopedia' chapter] and the dress will easily get back into shape. It will look like your dress straps and your bra straps are one. I find people are always afraid to 'stitch themselves' into clothing, but it is not frightening. Often a quick one, two with a needle and thread can make all the difference and remove the need for fidgeting.

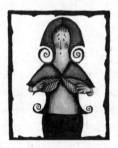

I enjoy wearing T-shirts, but as I get older my boobs shrink and my nipples seem to stick out more and are visible under some tops. Can you recommend one with smooth line (no seams) but thick enough to mask the nipple? – *Henrietta, Devon*

The other day at a friend's party, I noticed that my friend Alex's bosoms looked incredibly pert under a chiffon top. So I said, 'Alex, your breasts look incredibly perky. What's up?' It transpired that she had two Gossard Glossies sheer bras on, because, she said, it stopped her nipps showing. It worked, but you might find this a) extreme and b) expensive. What she didn't know is that Gossard Glossies do an opaque bra (£17.50 for the underwired bra, different shades available) which stops you having nipple show-through and is seamless. They are available in loads of places; call 01525 851122. Warners also do a great range called Not So Innocent Nudes. They have an underwired bra, £17, 32B–36D, which comes in toffee and body beige, and a double-ply underwired bra in the same colours and sizes 34B–36DD. Call 01159 795796 for stockists near you.

I had a baby by Caesarean six months ago and have seen my skirt size go from 12 to 16. I have a number of outfits which still fit my top half, but not at the bottom. I don't like exercise or dieting, so a friend suggested a panty girdle or control-top tights. I have tried control briefs and they are some help. I don't mind a bit of discomfort in the pursuit of fashion and have had a look at a girdle, but am not sure which one is best to flatter my tummy. Can you make any suggestions? (Playtex '18 hour'?) – *J. Morgan*

You didn't put an address so I have no idea where you are. Yes, well, who does like exercise or dieting, eh? But I have to say that sit-ups do help, and one can do these while watching telly, or even eating crisps, or even smoking (*Smoke and Stretch*, my new video, out soon). I do think a girdle would be best for you. I hate them, as I feel constricted in them, but if you don't mind a bit of discomfort then these will give the best results. Good old Playtex of those famous 18-hour-promise ads do have a good selection of panty girdles with high waists or lower waists. They really strap you in and provide firm control on the tummy. Prices start at £22.50 and range up to £35; call 01483 291450 for your nearest stockist (Johnny Loulou have the 18-hour waist girdle [style no. 2697], £25.50, and the 18-hour panty girdle [style no. 2690], £24.50, available from selected branches; enquiries 0171 629 7711). And Marks & Spencer also have a wide selection of control underwear, from thigh slimmers and waist slimmers (which claim to take 2" off the waist!) to tummy slimmers in their Smooth Line range. Prices start at £6.50 from branches nationwide (0171 935 4422). Damart also have a selection of pantie girdles from £7.99 (which my mum swears by, she won't have any others). To order a catalogue call 01274 510000. Control-top tights are OK (and just about everyone does a pair, though I've yet to find one brand radically better than another), but they won't really hold you in in the way you seem to want.

Can you help me with the address of an old-fashioned corsetière? It's really for my husband, who has had an operation which has left him without much in the way of stomach muscles – currently he is wearing a wide elastic belt from John Bell and Croydon because he hates all the things designed by the hospital and says they are useless. He knows just what he wants and thinks someone with the necessary skills could make it for him. I realize this is probably too odd a request to find its way into your column, but there might be other people who need a good corset made to measure for other reasons. – *Sue Davies, Bucks*

Nothing is too odd a request to be answered. Ready? Try surgical
appliance manufacturer BLS Healthcare Limited, who are at 49
Gregory Boulevard, Nottingham, tel: 0115 9780569. Axfords in
Brighton (01273 327944) and Vollers in Portsmouth (01705 799030)
do mail-order ready-made corsets. One of my readers tells me that
M. P. Garrod, 43 Emmbrook Road, Wokingham, Berks RG41 1HG,
fax: 01189 785577, though expensive, offers superb workmanship. I.
P. Norris, 114 Church Green Road, Bletchley, Milton Keynes MK3
6DD, is described by the same reader (J.L. from California, hi!) as
offering 'very good work, reasonably priced'; Jenyns Orthopaedics
in Sydney, New South Wales, Australia (well . . . you never know)
is 'well made but expensive'.

**My sister is partially sighted and we are both elderly and live 100-odd
miles apart. For a number of years I have bought her bras for her – size 32C
Triumph Doreen, made of cotton. This is no longer made. Harways have a
cross-over style but she would like a bra similar to the one she used to
have. – *Joy, Spalding, Lincs***

Well, did I find out a lot about the Doreen bra, a staple for many a
year of the bigger-bosom woman! OK, then, Joy, you have your
Doreen and your Doreen Cotton. The Doreen Cotton in 32C has
indeed been discontinued; it started at a size 34C. The Doreen starts
at 32B; in 34 it starts at C cup (and it goes up to a 50F). But wait!
Triumph have another one in the same shape but it's called the
Gracita + Cotton and it has a higher cotton content than the
Doreen Cotton (which had 25 per cent cotton); the Gracita has 35
per cent cotton and it's £2 cheaper at £18! Are you still with me,
Joy? The difference lies in the finish: the Gracita is much prettier
and has more lace. The aforementioned Gracita is a soft (as
opposed to underwired) bra, like the original Doreen Cotton was.
But if you're interested, the Gracita + Cotton R is underwired,
costs £21 and is made of a spanking 50 per cent cotton. How's
about that, then? Triumph enquiries should be made to 01793
720232. They'll tell you your nearest stockist, but they said that
Harways can get it in. If you have any problems at all getting it,
then write back to me and I'll try to get you one direct from Triumph (this personal service is only for you, Joy, because I think
you sound nice, buying your sister's bras for her).

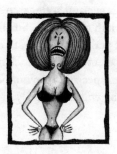

I am a 5'2" size 8 with a 32DD bust. It's an absolute nightmare. On the extremely rare occasions when I have found something that fits me well, people are amazed to discover my 'great' figure. However, most of the time I feel a freak quite honestly. I have two problems: clothes and bras. I discovered Bravissimo through your column but was disappointed to find the range in 32DD extremely limited. The only bra in a 32DD in my local M&S is 'minimizer'. Horrid – it was depressing to have my shape flattened, especially since I have worked hard on accepting my size. Clothes are becoming a real issue, especially with forthcoming weddings and an image at work to keep up. Is there a mail-order catalogue which specializes in petite sizes, and separates in particular? I have tried all the retail petite ranges but am disappointed by the limited range. To add to the trouble, not everyone seems to be aware that when you are small but short, hems and sleeves have to be scaled down accordingly. M&S are the exception, but the choice is not great. Please help! – _Nuala Murray, Edinburgh_

Well, first a little pep talk about bosoms. Mine seem to have gone from a 36DD to a 34DD or even a bloody 32E in certain styles. You sound like you have a fabulous, and I mean bloody fabulous (I realize I am swearing a lot) figure. It is the rest of the world that is odd. This doesn't make it easier, I know. If you read my column regularly you will know that Bravissimo (07000 2442727) is only one of three solutions for gorgeous busts; Margaret Ann (01985 840520) and Bust Stop (0181 943 9733) are the other two. On to clothes: Little Women is a mail-order catalogue specifically for shorter women, with dress sizes from 6 to 20. They have twenty-five garments which are fairly classic (work and casual) and come in six/seven different fabrics. There is usually a choice of three different lengths for skirts, trousers and sleeves; tailored skirts come in six different lengths. The size 8 statistics are 32–24–34. Call 0117 9639588 for catalogue and mail order. Things are slowly but surely getting better for those with bosoms; there is more choice and styles aren't so 'surgical'. [Make sure you also have a look in the 'Big . . . Small' chapter for more tips on people who do good petites ranges. But you should also investigate the Dressmaker's Directory at the back of the book and look into having things made especially for you. Not as expensive as you may think and everything will fit perfectly.]

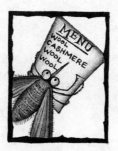

beasties under the bed
and what to do with them, as well as how to deal with stains and smelly things
moths, carpet beetles, sweaty stains and smelly feet

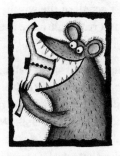

I have a horrible problem: my clothes have started getting tiny holes in them. I have put down so much moth repellent my wardrobe stinks. It's not only my knitwear they seem to be eating, but everything. What on earth can I do? – *Bettina Miller, Coventry*

I don't think you have moths at all. I think you have woolly bears, a.k.a. carpet beetles. You do not even need a carpet to warrant a visit from these pests. The bad news is that they are incredibly difficult to get rid of. The good news is that at least you don't have rats or cockroaches. Woolly bears shed their skin when they become adults (have you been finding tiny brown things that look like cocoons?) and the adults look like rolled-up bogies (they are very small creatures). They love dust and crevices. Please try doing the following. You will need to wash or dry clean ALL your clothes. Thoroughly hoover your carpet or wash your floor – if it's wooden or lino – with a solution of Borax (household cleaner available from Boots). Use Borax to wash the insides of your drawers, cupboards, walls (everything – they hate Borax). Then get about ten spray cans of Doom (again from Boots or Johnny Loulou, tel: 0171 629 7711) and spray your carpet/floor, inside your cupboards, your shelves, curtains, etc., paying special attention to corners and crevices: follow the instructions on the can. When you put your clothes back, put jumpers in zip bags and cover any special clothes you have with plastic hanging bags. Lakeland Limited (015394 88100) and Johnny Loulou do these, and Lakeland also do great resealable bags that you can put single items in. They are called zipper bags (medium is ref. no. 1725 and a pack of twenty-five costs £5.75; and large is ref. no. 1726 and costs £3.95 for ten). Or you can try their See Through Storage Bags (ref. no. 1893, £5.95 for fifteen), which are like big bin bags, but you can see through them. They also do lots of other storage items to cover clothes with, under-the-bed storage, etc. This will ensure that if you didn't get all of the woolly bears, at least you can limit the damage. This is a real nightmare problem to deal with, but there is no point being half-hearted about it. Good luck.

I am desperate to know how to stop moths eating my clothes. They have eaten their way through a surprising array of fabrics (including the felt covers of the piano hammers! and various rugs and fabric bags, not to mention silk shirts, velvet suits and all-wool jumpers!!). What can I do? I am paranoid that these hideous, dusty, flappy, useless creatures will devour my frocks and jumpers and nice shirts. So far I have been lucky and they haven't made their way to my room yet, but in the last three days I have found four of them in my wardrobe! I've seen the damage they wreak – please help. Do mothballs work? They smell so bad, I don't really want to go out with the lingering aroma of Eau de Naphthalene. I will do anything you suggest. – *Theresa Moore, Bristol*

Moths and carpet beetles [as previously mentioned] are on the increase. This is due to milder winters and the fact that we are just not as house-proud as our elders were . . . oh dear. I have had hundreds of similar enquiries, so this is for all of you. What you have to do is not dissimilar to the method for getting rid of woolly bears, so apologies for any repetition, but I like to be clear: first off, you have to wash/dry-clean your clothes, as this will kill the baby moths (and it is the grubs that do the damage, not the adults). Then you need to segregate your clothes as much as possible. This is to limit damage, so that if one thing gets reinfested the whole lot won't. You need to do this for drawers, wardrobes, chests, etc., either by using zipped plastic bags or zipped hanging bags [see previous problem]. Very precious things should be kept to one a bag. Then buy some very fine muslin (not expensive) and cut it into squares into which you put moth powder if you can find it; if not, put some mothballs in a heavy-duty plastic bag and scrunch them up with a rolling pin (do not let the rolling pin come into contact with the moth stuff as this is not healthy!) and tie it up with some string so it looks like a bouquet garni (don't get them muddled up or you will have some queer-tasting soups). Throw a couple of these little bundles into each zipper bag/hang them from hangers here and there/drop them into drawers. Then get some Vapona or Secto moth killers (Sainsbury's, Boots, Johnny Loulou) and hang a couple off the rail in your wardrobe. These don't smell and are clean and easy, but you will have to change them every six months.

Now for things like curtains, carpets and piano keys: buy some cans of the delightfully named Doom (Boots, Johnny Loulou) and spray them, following the instructions. You will need to renew all applications every six months but I think you'll find they bother you no more. Good night.

With the change of seasons, I would love to put my winter clothes away for a few months. This would free up more cupboard and hanging space and would give the clothes a proper 'rest'. Can you suggest an easy and not too expensive way to store clothes for a few months? Hopefully something that will keep them safe from insects and smelling fresh rather than musty when they are eventually unpacked. Any suggestions would be gratefully received. – *Marilyn Garces, London*

Well, this reply comes from Dawna Walter, who is the founder of the Holding Company, which specializes in all sorts of groovy ways to store things (find them at 241–245 King's Road, London sw3 5el, enquiries and mail order: 0171 610 9160): 'When storing winter clothing the most important thing is to make sure everything has been either washed or dry-cleaned, as moths feast on remnants of leftover food and other debris. Everything should be removed from plastic coverings such as dry-cleaners' bags, as they yellow light-coloured fabrics. I would always advise neatly folding all your clothing and placing them in under-bed storage bags made of cotton. These allow the clothes to breathe and keep insects out. An alternative is a well-constructed cardboard box with a tight-fitting lid. Please be certain that this is a damp-free environment. If there is a chance of damp or any humidity, I would use plastic storage boxes or under-bed clear plastic bags. I would add a packet of silica gel, which is commonly used as a dehumidifier in most packages and should be available from a good hardware store.' [Also see my tips for dealing with moths.]

I am so embarrassed about my question I am going to sign this letter with a pseudonym – my problem is sweat stains on clothes which I simply cannot remove. I am not a particularly sweaty person and I never wear things more than once before they are washed, yet this problem seems insoluble. I never used to find this a problem and I am wondering whether it is the deodorants I use that are the source of the difficulty. It seems worst with pure silk and fine polyester fabrics. I would be so grateful for your advice on which deodorant to use to avoid the problem. – *Elsie, Harlow*

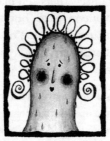

Don't be embarrassed, Elsie, we all sweat. Sweat is secreted from the apocrine glands and contains lipids, ammonium compounds, reducing sugars and salts. Some of the components of deodorants are aluminium salts. These can fix the lipids to the fabric surface, making their removal more difficult and allowing the yellowing/ darkening effect (which always occurs when unsaturated lipids are exposed to the atmosphere for any period) to occur. Also, some aluminium salts can hydrolyse to give an acidic solution. This acidic solution can transfer from the skin to clothing, resulting in damage to the fabric. Fancy stuff, eh? And just to make things even more difficult, the stains could be from your sweat or your antiperspirant/deodorant! But whatever they are from, all difficult stains benefit from having detergent applied directly to them before washing, as well as the stain-removal spray you are using. You could also try ACE, which is a very gentle bleach and is good for all sorts of stain removal, even on delicates. It may also be that the silk/polyester fabric absorbs the sweat more easily and stains more because the fabric you mention tends to be thinner and more deli- cate. I was going to suggest soaking the affected area in clear vine- gar, which is great for removing all stains, but I haven't tried this yet, so proceed with caution. But a most helpful man from Birm- ingham wrote in to suggest this: 'The best thing to remove sweat stains is a solution of sodium percarbonate at the fabric's max. tem- perature. It is a high-oxygen, chlorine-free bleach which is found in many stain removers and some fabric whiteners. It is fairly harm- less stuff, if you can get it from someone who works in a lab of any sort all the better. The best way to remove antiperspirant stains is a solution of citric acid, again as hot as the fabric will tolerate. You can buy citric acid from the shops that supply home brewers, or you can ask your pharmacist to get you some. Again it is fairly harmless stuff; I think it works best with aluminium-based stains.'

My boyfriend has unbearably smelly feet. This is a shame since he has beautiful taste in footwear, wearing bespoke brogues for work, but at home he wears trainers. I am unsure if the trainers are causing the problems because all his shoes smell. He won't think of wearing special insoles or anything like that. What can I do? – *A. Ellis (Ms), Penzance*

This is a problem I sympathize with, having had a boyfriend whose feet smelt so bad I thought there was going to be a ghostly manifestation every time he took his shoes off. I guess you know about the alternating shoes theory: i.e., giving your shoes a day off every other day so they have a chance to rest and the pong doesn't build up. Johnny Loulou do fabulous cedar-wood shoe trees, £26 a pair, which will not only keep your shoes in shape (very important for leather shoes) but also impregnate them with a nice cedar-wood smell. The Holding Company (0171 610 9160) [as mentioned already in this chapter], also make them for the slightly cheaper price of £24.50. Lakeland Limited (015394 88100) make Fragrant Clothes Fresheners that look like little tea-bags and are filled with herbs and spices (also good for repelling insects); they cost £3.95 for a pack of twenty-five. The other option worth trying for the trainers is washing them (if they are washable) in vodka, said to neutralize all nasty whiffs. This is an old wives' tale I have never tried on trainers and I would be interested to know if it works. Tell him to be careful dropping his cigarette butts, though – a smelly-footed boyfriend is a drag; a spontaneously combusting one is momentarily amusing but ultimately not to be recommended.

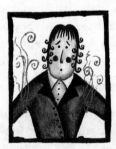

This is a very embarrassing problem so PLEASE do not print my name! However, it must be a common problem for the million other commuters who endure the same overheated trains as me through the winter, so I wish I had the courage to own up, but I don't . . . Is there anything you can do to get rid of a sweaty smell once it has got into a jacket? It happens like this: it's

freezing cold outside, you get into an overheated train, you sweat like mad
for twenty minutes, then you get out and it's cold again. Apart from developing every virus under the sun, much worse is that your dry-clean-only jacket
is smelly. You send it to the cleaners and lo! – it comes back all fresh and
sweet-smelling. However, the slightest bit of warmth, even the application
of a warm iron, brings the problem back with a vengeance. There seems to
be nothing on earth that will get rid of it. Annie, I know you will have the
answer, please! – *Mrs Elizabeth May Phillips, Potters Lane, Derby*

Oh, whoops! Forgot to leave your name off and now everyone
knows! Only joking, readers, the real identity of this sweet lady is
well shielded by me and Mrs E.M.P. of P.L., Derby, is but a fig-
ment of my imagination. I spoke to a lovely man called David, who
is a garment-analysis technician at the Fabric Care Research Association, and he said that in general cleaning has limits and sometimes things have just had it. Dry-cleaning is a process which is
good for creases and dirt removal but not really for getting rid of
odours. Washing is much better for smells, so if you can, wash it.
What I suggest you try here is sponging: put a sponge in a solution
of water and clothes washing liquid (like Woolite), as if you were
hand-washing, and add about half a capful of white or clear vinegar
or vodka to the solution as well – vinegar or vodka is very good for
neutralizing smells (but please do a patch test first!). Wring the
sponge out and dab on the affected area a few times and then rinse
in the same way. There is also a dry-cleaning process called ozone-
cleaning method which is quite specialized – it's often used on
smoke-damaged garments, though usually on household textiles
rather than clothes. What happens is, the garment is put into an
ozone chamber and this is good for getting rid of odours; however,
I don't know of anywhere that does it and nor did David.

A reader called Micky wrote in with some very useful advice:

With reference to your spurious Mrs Phillips's problem. At the Ideal Home
Exhibition last year I bought a product called Fresh Again for uniforms and
costumes (it costs £2.95 plus p&p for a small pump-action spray which
apparently lasts ages). The company importing it from America is called
Upstage Theatrical Dry Cleaners of Unit 8, Acorn Production Centre, 105
Blundell Street, London N7 9DW, tel: 0171 609 9119 (evening answerphone
0181 207 6436). I have used it on my favourite leather jacket with great success – apparently it was used on the jackets worn in *Grease*. There are other

variants that I use, one for smelly trainers (!) and another, oh glory, to get rid of the smell of stale smoke. And no, I don't have any connection with the company (or with *Grease*, for that matter). – *Micky Gwilliam, London*

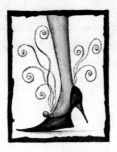

Smelly feet seem to run in my family, with four out of seven siblings suffering. Thankfully I'm not one of them! I told my sister about your column and agreed to write as she is too embarrassed. Her feet really stink, even washing them three times a day and changing her socks. It's very distressing as she often has to wear nylon hose to the office (she's a lawyer) and this definitely makes it worse. Cotton/linen/silk isn't really that bad and we wondered if you knew of any supplier who made natural-fibre hose? She has found thick cotton tights but is looking for sheer hose or at least slightly opaque. Any suggestions would be greatly appreciated. – *Mary Evers, London*

I don't know about natural hosiery that is also very sheer but what I can suggest is that your smelly-footed siblings try Funn hosiery. They are a mail-order company who supply the film and stage trade with all sorts of hosey. They have a comprehensive range of silk and cotton (mostly stockings because tights need more stretch). They have about thirty-eight colours of cotton stockings – their stock is a little depleted (not every colour in every S, M and L size) but still pretty comprehensive. The more antique, unusual colours of seamed silk stockings can be expensive but ivory cotton stockings aren't a problem; they cost £4.95 (p&p included), sizes S, M and L, and they could always be dyed, I suppose. They also do something called Opera tights, which are 75 per cent cotton (which is on the inside), 20 per cent Supplex and 5 per cent Lycra, but they are very opaque. Anyway, Funn can be contacted by writing to PO Box 102, Steyning, West Sussex, BN44 3DS, with an SAE, and they will send a list of colours/sizes, etc. Fogal at 36 New Bond Street, London W1Y 9HD, tel: 0171 493 0900, do two types of cotton-mix tights. Fogal are extremely expensive, but then their products are of excellent quality. All the same, I'm not sure how many people could afford them – they do Carpi, which cost £100 and are 60 per cent cotton, 25 per cent silk and 15 per cent polymide (which is mostly in the waistband), in a range of about eight colours, including black; and Siestriere, which cost £92 and are 58 per cent cotton, 23 per cent silk and 19 per cent nylon, in the same range of colours. All in sizes S, M and L.

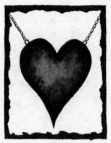

pane, amore e cha cha cha
this means 'bread, love and chitter-chatter'
in italian and this chapter is all about crafty
and useful tips, mostly learned in italy
*how to clean suede, get wax out of clothes
and chewing gum out of hair*

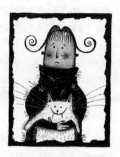

I wear a lot of black and am forever getting fluff on my clothes which looks awful. None of those brushes advertised as defluffers works. Is there any way to look well groomed? – *C. Forbes (Ms), Bristol*

You can get those contraptions that roll around and have replaceable sheets of stickiness, or those ones that are meant to 'reactivate' under the auspices of a good run under a cold tap. To my mind, they are all crap. The best, cheapest and only way to defluff is to get some good old parcel tape (sticky tape will do too, but parcel tape tends to be more adhesive and covers more square inches at a time). Take a length of tape and stick it round your hand and then just work your way over the garment. Easy-peasy and bloody cheap.

I have this wonderful cotton coat that I bought years ago. It's black cotton jersey and I wear it with everything. The problem is that I went to a dinner party and the hostess put my coat on a chair that was underneath a candle and now I have candle wax all over it. I've tried picking it off but it doesn't work. Should I wash it? – *Sue Paige, Southampton*

Sue the bloody stupid hostess. Damn nuisance. Nah, don't bother picking it off and don't wash it. What you do is put some brown paper over it and iron it. The wax will melt and be absorbed by the brown paper and will disappear from your beloved coat. Make sure the iron is clean (when it's cool) before you use it again and next time make sure the dippy hostess trying to re-create a scene from *Dracula* has a proper place to hang your coat. Damn nuisance.

I have a long white satin skirt that I love wearing but it is a bit see-through. I hate wearing G-strings and none of the skin-tone knickers I have tried seems 'thin' enough (you can still see the line of the knickers). Surely someone somewhere has done a gossamer-thin pair of briefs? – *Franca Malson, Bedford*

If you really feel that the range of skin-tone knickers that is currently on the market is not suitable (and M&S do an excellent selection), then try this: take two pairs of fine-denier tights, chop them off at mid-thigh and wear them instead of underwear. This is not recommended for everyday use (nylon next to your cha cha is not the healthiest thing) but it is an excellent solution to your problem and one used by stylists caught out on fashion shoots. Very unattractive to look at, so avoid high gales.

I am always getting make-up on my clothes as I pull the garment over my head. I can't always get dressed before applying make-up. What do you do? – *Emma Phillips, Barrow-in-Furness*
This isn't a problem I have as I have never managed to work out the difference between an eye pencil and a lip pencil. I even eat off my lip gloss, when I think to apply it. Sadly, between bringing up babies and running a pig farm, make-up has got lost along the way. But this is what models do on shoots, when make-up is always applied before dressing. Buy some synthetic georgette from your local department store, about half a metre. Then, put it over your head before you slip your clothes on. The georgette will protect your clothes but still allow you to get dressed easily (and still allow you to see – always handy to prevent claustrophobia attacks). If you're not too drunk when you get home, remember to do it when you get undressed too (although in reverse the process is more fiddly). Works like magic.

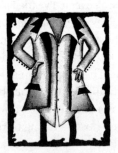

I like to wear shirts outside my trousers but find that when I wear a jacket on the way to work the shirt tails are always longer than the jacket. Should I make a feature of this or wear longer jackets? – *M. Donaghy (Mrs), Bath*
If you want to make a feature of the shirt tails you could also pull the shirt cuffs so that they peek out of the jacket sleeves and all this spillage looks intentional rather than just scruffy. You could buy a

longer-length jacket, but if your shirt tails are that long, to cover them you will end up with a very long jacket and looking like a Teddy boy. Is shortening the shirt not an option? But perhaps the simplest way is to get a length of thick, soft elastic, tying it into a circle, stepping into it so that it sits over you shirt and then pulling the shirt up until its hem sits comfortably above your jacket hem. When you reach your destination pull the shirt tails out of the elastic which remains discreetly about your waist awaiting the journey home.

What is the best way to get chewing gum out of clothes?
– Arantxa, Sutton Coldfield
You need to freeze the garment, then the gum will just snap off. Incidentally, if anyone ever gets chewing gum in their hair, a very nice man at Wrigley's told me the trick is either to get some cocoa butter (from chemists) and work it into the hair and then wash as normal (it dissolves the chewing gum), or, if you can't get hold of that, mix fat or butter with chocolate or cocoa powder (if necessary heat it up and then let it cool until it is still malleable but not hot) and then work the paste into the hair and wash. Rather handy trick, I thought. Thank you, Wrigley's.

My husband wears slip-on shoes and I hate them. He wears them with everything. He does know how to tie laces but seems to prefer the comfort of slip-ons. I know it's unfair of me to want him to change them, but is there any great fashion argument for not wearing slip-ons that I could try to persuade him with? *– Lindsay, Salisbury*
I would say it's unfair of you to try to change him, except for the fact that I agree with you, so go right ahead. The reason I despise slip-on shoes is because I think you can't trust a man who wears them. You know – easy on, easy off. What reason can you give him? As I have said before, with men the best way to get them to change anything is to say that what you like is a real turn-on: i.e., 'Darling, I get really turned on at the sight of black brogues,' etc. This works with everything and is so much better than nagging. I told my husband years ago that I got turned on at the sight of a man wearing rubber gloves and cleaning/doing the washing up. I've barely had to do either since.

Could you please give me some advice on caring for buck leather? I recently bought a pair of black ankle boots which I sprayed with matt leather dressing before I wore them, but now, after several wearings, they

have become a little marked and I should like to know the best way to keep them clean. – *Val Bardsley (Mrs), Norwich*

Buck, or nubuck, leather needs special care as it is more delicate and finer than conventional leather and suedes. You could try Meltonian's Suede and Nubuck Cleaning Block (£2.75), enquiries: 01753 523 971. It removes spots and stains and is suitable for any colour. When suede and nubuck become worn they are susceptible to shiny bald patches, just like tired old men, and this block restores texture (to shoes, not heads). What I do, though, is rub my nubuck and suede shoes very lightly with a fine sandpaper. On light-coloured suede/nubuck, I dust them with talc and then brush it off with a soft brush (I find babies' toothbrushes are ideal for this). If they're quite dirty, I hold the shoe over a steaming kettle and gently brush the pile with this soft brush; the steam cleans the suede/nubuck. On black suede or nubuck, nothing beats holding the shoe over a candle and brushing gently. This is what my mother used to do with all her fine suede stilettos as a youngster; the soot kind of rejuvenates black suede.

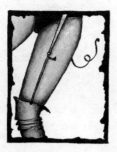

stockings and suspenders
plus boring stuff too about tights and socks
*where to get a six-strap suspender belt,
silk socks and pregnancy tights*

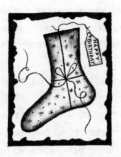

It is my husband's birthday soon and he is really boring. All he likes are socks. This would seem easy, but I just can't buy him any old pair, it doesn't seem like a present. Are there any super-special ones on the market I could buy for him? – *Tina Edmonds (Mrs), Ipswich*

There are, but they cost. Pantherella do cashmere socks. They are extremely soft and luxurious and have 10 per cent nylon in them for added strength (cashmere on its own is lovely but doesn't stand up to wear and tear very well). They cost from £44.95 in various colours and patterns and two lengths from department stores nationwide (call 0116 283 1111 for a stockist near you). Apparently some men swear by them and once they've got a pair of Pantherella's on their feet won't go back to anything else. This could be an expensive business. Be warned.

I enjoy wearing fully fashioned seamed stockings with suspenders for their feel and glamorous looks. However, it is difficult to keep the seams straight over a long period and there is nothing worse than crooked seams for ruining the glamorous effect. Do you have any useful advice? A suspender belt with six straps might help but does anyone manufacture such a thing? – *G. Roper (Mrs), Peterborough, Cambs*

Yes, I do know someone who makes a six-strap suspender thing and that will help keep your seams straight, but just before I launch into that let me say that what will also help is if you wear a 'deep' suspender belt, i.e., one that has a substantial piece of material to it that really anchors the s/b to your hips and not one that is just a flimsy strip of material. Now then, try Cover Girl Shoes, 44 Cross Street, London N1 2BA, tel: 0171 354 2883. This is ostensibly a shop for transvestites but they are very helpful and sell six-strap suspender belts with metal clasps for about £25.

I have a very annoying problem. *All* my tights give at the seams, even at the

first wear! I am 5'5", with my widest point (at the top of my thighs) approx.
41". I weigh just under ten stone and normally wear size 14 skirts. I have tried
nail varnish on a new tear but it makes it worse. What would you suggest?
– *Helen, London*

I am not sure what you mean by 'they give at the seams' as most
tights do not have seams other than around the top. Is this where
they give? First, look for tights with Lycra in them. This fibre has
'stretch and recover' properties and for hosiery manufacturers to be
able to include Lycra in their product, DuPont (Lycra's manufacturers) insist that the tights meet various criteria – such as having a
gusset. A gusset on tights ensures that you can walk without pulling
on the seams too much. You are not fat, so that is not causing the
problem (in any case, tights, like condoms, are miraculous things
that stretch beyond all imagination). Having said that, are you sure
you are buying tights that are big enough for you? I always find that
people buy tights too small for them, somehow thinking that 'large'
is for people who are six foot tall. I never buy smaller than a
medium, even though according to the packet size-guide I should be
buying small. But getting them in a size bigger means you don't
have to pull on them so much. Nail varnish should work – you need
to apply it to the bottom and top of a new tear, although this is only
a temporary measure. I wear mostly Wolford as I think their quality
is superb, especially their opaques, some of which I've had for years.
You might also like to pop down to Fogal, in London, with stores
in Sloane Street and New Bond Street. They make very expensive
and very good hosiery and are also most knowledgeable.

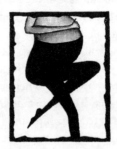

I am pregnant and am finding it harder and harder to find tights to fit me. I
was by no means large before and am hardly huge now, but even extra-
large tights are getting snug on me. Does anyone do really big tights?
– *Mary Lonsdale, London*

Yes, people do extra-big tights – Hue do a Queen Size pair for women with more to grab hold of – but that's not what you need. You need maternity tights, which are specially shaped to accommodate your bump. Hue also do some, which cost from £9.95, as do Mothercare, who have a value pack of three 15-denier pairs in black, navy and natural – they cost from £4.25 a pack (sizes 1, 2). You really should be wearing these and not just huge tights! Blooming Marvellous do packs of two in mink, black or navy for £5.99, and also opaques in black or navy, £6.99 for a two-pack, one size. Enquiries and mail order: 0181 391 4822.

As a chilblain sufferer, I find the only solution is either to look like Scott of the Antarctic or wear real-wool tights. A few years ago these were really popular and easy to find. I have found only one make of wool-rich tights in my local store – from a Finnish company, Kymen Sukka Oy – but these sell out of my size (large) very early in the season and the store has not been overly helpful in reordering. Your help would make next winter a pleasure rather than a pain. – *Sylvia Fox (Mrs), Poole*

Try silk socks, which are renowned for keeping feet warm. The Innovations catalogue do some, in two lengths, in black, cream or blue, costing £9.95 (call 0990 807060). They are thin enough to wear *with* your tights. I too used to have a thing for high-content wool tights, but they aren't the best for warmth, comfort, or fit – woollen tights grow with body heat and bag at the ankles – so please don't discount blends. I once had a number for Kymen Sukka Oy but it is no longer valid and all attempts to locate a new one have failed. Fogal have done some wonderful ones and, before you scream at the prices, believe me, the initial outlay is worth it. Kashmir, £200, which is 50 per cent silk, 40 per cent cashmere and 10 per cent nylon, sizes S, M and L; Nepal, 80 per cent wool, 10 per cent cashmere and 10 per cent nylon, price £94, sizes S, M and L. Yes, of course I realize that this is a huge amount of money, but I'm just giving you the information. Fogal are based in London, with stores in New Bond Street and Sloane Street, and they do mail order (but not a catalogue), tel: 0171 493 0900. Fogal also do thick cotton tights with Lycra (much cheaper), which they assure me will keep you warm. Cheaper and still excellent, Wolford do a woollen-blend pair (about 60 per cent wool) for £22 from department stores (call 0171 935 9202 for stockists).

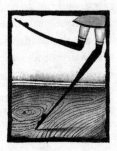

I've been trying to get hold of a pair of black over-the-knee socks but to no avail. I am desperate to get hold of a pair as I have got quite nice legs and they will look very sexy with my miniskirt. I know they were all the rage about twelve months ago but no one seems to sell them/wear them any more. Please help. – *Julia, Salisbury*

Johnny Loulou still do them, two types: a wool/Lycra mix (called Jonelle) for £3.45 and a cotton mix called the KS, £3.95 (enquiries: 0171 629 7711).

Your advice about shoulder pads and see-through blouses inspired me to write in [see 'Can I, Should I?' chapter]. Do you also consider it tacky for me to show the 'bumps' of my suspenders when wearing a straight skirt? I have been a dedicated wearer of stockings and suspenders for about twenty-five years, even before they became fashionable, and latterly afterwards too. I don't wear skin-tight skirts and always ensure that I wear a slip or that they are lined. A short time ago, when suspenders were very much in fashion, we all couldn't help showing our bumps, but now that stockings aren't so widely worn I feel rather out on a limb. So what do you think, am I the strumpet that some of my friends say I am? – *Shelly, Wilmslow*

The wearing of suspenders does not *make* you a strumpet, Shelly. This involves other things, such as the frequent and sometimes inappropriate removal of one's pants in the company of surname-not-known gentlemen. If you don't wear skin-tight skirts and/or wear a slip or lined skirt, then the bumps of your suspenders won't show *that* much, surely? A hint of suspender is rather nice, I think. I know what you mean, though. I love wearing stockings and suspenders, but only dare do so with a particular skirt that is long, lined and of fairly thick crêpe. Then it is only obvious that I am wearing them when I sit on my husband's lap (or anyone else's, if I am very drunk). I should continue with your sensible use of them – and your friends are obviously jealous, because we all know that stockings and suspenders are by far the sexiest form of hosiery, it's just that most of us can't be figged to wear them.

My daughters and I have always followed Marlene Dietrich's advice (does any girl today know who that glamour queen was?) to wear shoes as close as possible to the skin tone of the leg, for a longer, slimmer silhouette. It lifts short girls and slims plump girls and is easy on the purse because the 'long naked leg' illusion matches red, blue, green and even black. –
Magda, Gibraltar

Thanks, Magda, for your words of Gibraltarian wisdom, although I disagree with you on the source of this advice – I think it was Marilyn Monroe. You are right, though, that wearing skin-tone shoes does indeed make your legs look longer (obviously you need to wear skin-tone hosiery, too, if you cannot go bare-legged), but they aren't quite as versatile as you make out. If your skin tone is of the pinky-beige variety, then wearing matching shoes will not really go with dark suits; I think it looks naff and odd. It is ideal, however, for summer wear or if you are wearing an outfit of a difficult colour (i.e., turquoise or yellow), as buying matching shoes for such a garment would be difficult.

I adore coloured stockings: greens, blues, purples, pinks, yellows and rusts. Dior used to do a really wide range of colours, but now I can't find them anywhere. They were such fun, can you help?
– Jo Haxby, Newmarket, Suffolk

Dior still do twenty colours of Diorella 15-denier stockings, which retail at about £1.95 a pair. It may just be that your local department store has narrowed down the range of colours it stocks. What you can do is either ask your local store to order the colours you want (and they should do this if they are good) or contact Christian Dior hosiery direct on 01455 272 322.

I am wondering whether you know where I can buy seamed tights? I have tried many places and can only buy stay-ups or stockings. Sock Shop, Wolford, John Lewis: no joy. – Rebecca Caroe, Maidenhead, Berkshire

Oh dear, readers. I am not feeling myself. In fact no one is feeling me, as my husband has had to go abroad to write and won't be back until Christmas and I am very sad and lost without him. There are only remnants of his scent on his fine woollen sweaters.

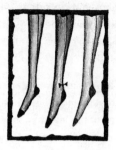

Sniff. Anyway, I must press on to bring fashion order into the world. Well, seamed tights do seem to be a bit thin on the ground, but here's who's done some: Couture (01455 272322), with point heel (that funny-looking thing in seamed tights that points up the ankle before becoming a seam), 15 denier with Lycra in black or fouine (brown), £4.99; and Oroblu (0181 743 4243), Riga, 20 denier with 15 per cent Lycra in black, natural, chocolate and blue/black, price £9.99. Both of these are available from stores nationwide, but I've put the enquiry number in so you can phone and get a stockist near you. John Lewis branches *do* sell a make called Melas, which has a seam and pointed heel, £3.45, in black, barely black, navy and natural.

I am a size 16–18 and have difficulty finding stockings that fit well. All of the stockings that I have tried run short, and the tops finish halfway up my thigh, making them difficult to secure to suspenders. I have tried a variety of brands in their 'Large' size without success. Can you please help? Thanks and regards. – *Jackie, Kent*

Independence Ltd (0181 861 1722 for mail order) have extra-long stockings in 20 and 30 denier in honey or mink, £6.50 for three pairs, £10.99 for six pairs. And Magnus (tel: 01604 831271), who also make shoes in larger sizes [see 'Big Shoe' directory] also sell extra-long stockings and tights which fit up to a size 22. Evans do both stockings and tights in their branches nationwide (enquiries: 0171 291 2405). Stockings come in natural or black, £3.50, and are one size. In tights there is a good selection, including glossies, run-resistant, sheer and opaques in winter. They start at £3.50 and they begin at 12 denier, in three sizes: 48", 52" and 60" hips. [Also make sure you read my advice about six-strap suspenders earlier in this chapter.]

Please help! I used to buy tights with a gusset gap ('airflow tights') which let the body breathe, so there was no odour. I got these from Tytex/Better

Living mail order, but they seem to have closed down or moved. Can I get such tights anywhere? If your information scouts could come up with a source I'd be very grateful. – *Sarah V., Athens*

Well, your letter came on hotel paper from a five-star hotel in Athens (fancy), so I can only assume you actually live in the UK. (I am flattered that on holiday you thought to write to me . . .) One tip is to cut the diamond gusset shape carefully out of a 'normal' pair of tights to allow for extra ventilation, or you could try Bhs's Body-Free tights, £5 for three (enquiries: 0171 262 3288). And Priory Healthcare do some (from £6.45 for four pairs + p&p; 01438 798 206), as do Aldrex (from £6.99 for three; write to Aldrex, Dept ALD 1021, Brandlesholme Road, Bury BL8 1BG or call 0161 236 5555 for a catalogue). Finally, try Woman in Mind (01204 525 115), who make all sorts of hosiery (Ventights, Open Crotch Tights) and whose priority is making sure there is a supply of fresh air to your cha cha.

I detest the demarcation line inflicted on the waist by tights. This is particularly alarming when one is wearing form-fitting evening wear. When last in New York I purchased two 'body stockings' from Victoria's Secret. They are like tights in that they have feet but they continue beyond the waistline to the chest and have little shoulder straps – a head-to-toe all-in-one. The only problem is that the body stockings I purchased are virtually opaque. I am looking for relatively sheer versions (in black) of the same beast. I have tried M&S with no success. In the past (in Canada) I have found a fishnet version in a sex shop. Not surprisingly, it was crotchless, which proved to be a blessing after a great deal of wine. However, I have not found the same relief in Soho. Please help me. I cannot believe that there are no body stockings in the fashion centre of the world. The success or failure of my Christmas season rests entirely on your worthy shoulders. Thank you very much. P.S. I do hope everything is well with you and, no, I am not insane. – *Siobhan, via e-mail*

Au contraire, Siobhan, you are quite insane. The crotchlessness came in handy after a great deal of wine? What do you mean? That you had relations with boys? That you were able to go '*faire pee-pee*' without having to remove your knickers? For your own sake, I have not printed your surname, or I fear you would be inundated with saucy enquiries from certain members of the community for whom the word crotchless is almost too much to bear, let alone when it rubs shoulders with words such as body stockings, fishnet, sheer, sex shop, Soho, beast and Canada. Let me help you. In the

'Index Extra' catalogue (page 264) there is exactly the thing: it is crotchless (I did not purposely seek out that it had this feature, it just coincidentally did; I think actually it is a pretty useful thing, as you said, otherwise you'd have to get completely undressed to go to the toilet) and seamless, with little shoulder straps. It's one size and fits up to 42" hips. It is nylon and black (though it has a little flower pattern on it). It's imaginatively entitled 'body stocking DV 049G' and costs £9. What a bargain. Call 0800 401080, lines open 7 a.m.–11 p.m., every day. Incidentally, Victoria's Secret haven't got one in their current catalogue but they do lots of brilliant things, so anyone interested should call 001 614 3375122.

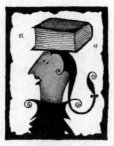

encyclopedia
maybe things you never knew
like the difference between a fibre and a fabric,
and whether silk worms lead happy lives

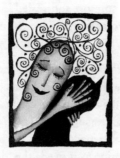

I recently purchased a blouse in Germany made of 100 per cent cupro. Is this a new fabric/fibre? It's quite wonderful – looks and feels like silk of a heavier quality. It should be hand-washed, which I have now done on a number of occasions, and ironing is a dream. It's silk without all the hard work. I do hope you can satisfy my curiosity. – *Meredity Brooks, Düsseldorf*

Cupro is the generic term for cuprammonium rayon (thank goodness) – basically just another type of rayon. It is a fibre and has been around for a long time, at least thirty years. Rayon is a fab fibre and can be made into various thicknesses. One of my favourite suits was a beige rayon one by Fenn Wright & Manson. It was fluid and gorgeous and got comments wherever I went. Foolishly, however, I started putting it in the washing machine (I rarely hand-wash, my hands weren't made to scrub) to save on dry-cleaning bills and it shrunk and shrunk until it was almost no more. It creased a lot, but ironed easily, like you said. I hope your curiosity is satisfied, Meredity, but remember it killed the Katze.

How do I iron a shirt properly? – *Mr Lewis, Bayswater*
I defer to an expert for this. A spokesman for London's premier dry-cleaners, Tothills, advises: 'First, use a good padded ironing board and a fine-mist water sprayer in addition to a steam iron. Start with the collar, then the cuffs, then the sleeves. [This prevents the shirt from being crushed, if you do the collar last, for example, you will crease the rest of the shirt.] Then, with the shirt unbuttoned and the button side facing upwards, iron the body of the shirt, working the fabric away from you as you iron. And always check the temperature of the iron is suitable for the shirt.' His branch alone handles some 600–800 shirts a week, more shirts than I ever plan to iron in a lifetime. For £4.10 a shirt, Tothills will launder and hand-iron your shirt and you will get it back either hung on a tissue-padded hanger or beautifully folded with tissue

paper, cardboard neck support and sealed in a cellophane bag. Cheap at the price, if you ask me. Express service costs extra and collection and delivery are available; call 0171 252 0100.

I have a linen jacket, which creases so easily I find it really difficult to iron flat, especially around the shoulders, and I end up with a crease along the shoulder pads and down the arms. Where can I buy a steamer that I could use while the jacket is on the hanger? – *William Peters, Aberdeen*
Really good industrial steamers are expensive and, anyway, linen benefits more from ironing as it needs the 'pressure' of an iron to give it that nice crisp look. What you could do is this: roll up a towel so that it fits into the length of the sleeve, then iron around the sleeves (rolling the sleeve as you go along). This doesn't give you creases down the arms because the towel provides a soft base (I find this easier than a sleeve board, because they never seem long or thin enough so you still end up with the creases). Then wrap the towel around your hand and iron the shoulders against your hand, effectively ironing in 3D. This is a very easy way of ironing all sorts of garments around the shoulders, which is always a tricky bit to do, especially with tailoring.

Having recently graduated, I now have a job that requires ties to be worn. Although I enjoy wearing ties, I have difficulty in getting the knot firm at the neck. No matter how I tie it, or what material they are made of, there is invariably a flash of shirt and top button between neck and knot. What am I doing wrong? – *Marten Hutt, Hertford College, Oxford*
I suspect that you are tying your tie in a 'four-in-hand knot', the easiest and most common way to knot a tie. A more complicated knot, but one that gives a better shape and hardly slips, is the Windsor. It is very hard to describe how to do this and in the column I said people could write in and get a printed sheet that shows you how to tie such knots as the four-in-hand, Prince Albert, Ascot cravat, etc. It's nothing fancy, but if anyone wants a copy, write to me c/o annie, Independent on Sunday, 1 Canada Square, London E14 5DL, and I'll send it (please enclose a SAE).

I keep reading about 'tonic' jackets, skirts and trousers. What is that exactly? – *Sandra, Kendal*
It means the fabric has a slight sheen to it and is slightly 'two tone' in the sense that it seems to change colour as the light on it moves.

It is very subtle and jolly nice, although not madly fashionable any more. I do like them, but only a few men can get away with tonic suits. My lovely husband is one of them.

As a vegetarian I try to be aware of how things are produced. I have a problem with silk – having heard it is produced by steaming silkworms alive; for years I avoided buying silk clothes. Can you tell me what goes on? I secretly hope that the silkworms have a happy little life, so I can buy silk with a clear conscience! – *Debbie Watson, Leeds*

Oh my dear. I rang the wonderful Textile Institute in Manchester, who told me that it *is* true. The silkworms' cocoons are killed by steam or hot air, then placed in hot water to soften the gum (known as sericin) which binds the silk to the cocoon. I didn't know this either and have to admit that I now look at silk in a different way. You will have to continue avoiding silk clothes if you feel this strongly about it. However, you may wish to consider Tencel, which is a good silk alternative. It is a cellulosic fibre which is kinder to the environment than the process to make viscose rayon is (in fact it was invented by Courtaulds for just that reason – because it was kinder). It is still a relatively new fibre (its generic name is lyocell, so you may see that in labels in the same way that you see Lycra's generic, elastane) and quite magnificent. It doesn't involve cruelty to animals in any way and is in fact extremely eco-friendly (if you're interested, it is made in a 'closed loop' system, which means that nothing gets out, although the chemical used to dissolve the cellulose is harmless anyway). Lots of people do it now in their collections; look for the swing ticket.

This letter caused a bit of a stir among readers. In order to help those of you who have had trouble sleeping since the Stephen King-like revelation that silkworms are boiled alive, I should like to print extracts from two letters:

The silkworm (larva) does live a very happy life and gorges itself for about twenty-eight days and nights on succulent white mulberry leaves. Having eaten enough, the larva makes a cocoon and goes to sleep. The larva then changes into a pupa, which remains dormant for about ten days. The cocoon can then be reeled immediately into a single silk filament, by submerging the cocoon in very hot water, which kills the pupa. The deceased pupa is not wasted but often used as either chicken or fish feed, and even sometimes consumed by the locals as a culinary delicacy. The only justification I can

offer about the demise of the silkworm pupa is that by continuing silk production many, many people are employed in developing countries.
– *Martin Hardingham, Textile Consultant, Somerset*

What about wild (tussah) silk? This is not as gorgeously smooth and shiny as reeled silk (when the silkworm is killed inside the cocoon so as not to break off any of the threads, and miles of continuous thread is produced), but it is obtained when the silkworm eats its way out of the cocoon, breaking the threads, which are then spun into yarn which is slightly rougher and less lustrous. – *Rachel Dufton, Winchester*

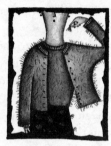

Is it true that keeping your jumpers in the fridge will stop angora from shedding? I am particularly interested because I have just been given a lovely angora twin-set. It's caramel-coloured, and all my black skirts and trousers are now black and caramel. Apart from this I wear contact lenses and all the fibres are a complete nightmare on the eyes. If the fridge is not the answer, what is? (I hope you do have an alternative, because my fridge is minuscule, and if cold temperatures are essential it may come to a choice between wearing my twin-set and eating.) – *Hester, Wimbledon*

I so sympathize. I was given a beautiful cashmere bouclé man's sweater from Joseph for Christmas once and it sheds everywhere. No scope for being unfaithful, I'd leave my trail, which is a shame as it's so cosy (in fact, when I was ill recently a friend rang up and coined the wonderful phrase 'Illness is always a bit better in a Joseph jumper'). I spoke to knitwear designer Rina Da Prato, who said that keeping jumpers in the fridge *does* stop them shedding, but you would have to keep returning them to the fridge to retain the effect (in an ideal world our jumper cupboards would be chilled, but this isn't an ideal world). We don't really know why, though. Rina also suggests using Woolite when washing and squeezing the jumper instead of wringing as this keeps the fibres from matting, then give it a light brush when dry. Unfortunately, there isn't a long-term solution (someone else suggested trying hairspray); there's obviously a great marketing opportunity here. Remember the best way to defluff your other clothes is to use parcel tape – boring, I know, but better than looking like you have been rolling in a sheep's pen. You shouldn't have to make a choice between food and fibres; chill your jumpers overnight, when maybe your fridge is less full.

I am constantly losing one half of sets of earrings and so have a box full of single earrings which I can't use but am fond of. Do you know of a jewellery maker who is willing to copy earrings exactly, and if so, how much is it likely to cost (they are not expensive jewels: for example, I have lost one of a marcasite pair, and another is moss agate and gold). – *Diana, Notting Hill*
This is a problem that a lot of people have, but I have to point out that copying *any* style of earring, even something cheap and mass-produced, is illegal. Having said this, your local jeweller will most probably be able to help you; you just have to pop in and ask. If you buy your earrings from a jewellery designer, however (and this doesn't necessarily mean expensive), they will almost always be able to make the lost earring again, as it's their design to do what they will with. If you remember where you got them from, it really is worth trying to trace the manufacturer and asking them, otherwise your local jeweller is your best bet. During the First World War it became popular to wear just one earring, as women had keepsakes (such as buttons) made into an earring to remind them of their husbands at war; this is where the fashion for just one earring (à la Human League) comes from.

How does one fold and securely fasten a sari? – *Judith Sawyer, London*
I spoke to Kiki Siddiqi (what a fantastic name, eh?) at Ritu, 16 North Audley Street, London w1y 1we, tel: 0171 491 4600, who make beautiful saris that range from £125 to £1,400. They would be only too happy to help you – or any newcomers to saris – drape your sari, as it is much easier to show than it is to explain in words. [Incidentally, Kiki gave me a sheet of easy diagrams on 'how to' which I can forward on to you, and anyone else interested, if you send me an SAE c/o annie, Independent on Sunday, 1 Canada Square, London e14 5dl, but really, there is no substitute for having an expert show you firsthand.] But in the meantime, this is what Kiki had to say: 'The sari is a piece of material

about six yards long and four wide. Most of this is pleated at the waist, wound round to form a skirt, and the remaining fabric is swept across the upper body to cover at least one shoulder and sometimes veiling the head. It is part of a three-piece ensemble of a blouse, snug and to the waist, and a full-length petticoat with drawstring waist. To wear your sari, hold it with the inner edge in the left hand and tuck it into the petticoat at the right hip. Take the sari round the back of your hip and tuck the upper border in as you go around the waistband of the petticoat until you get to the front again. Now pleat half to two-thirds of the sari – the pleats should be about four inches deep and overlapping, and then tucked into the petticoat waistband at the centre of the (front) body. This sounds more difficult than it is. The remaining fabric is passed round the left hip and then gathered or pleated again to drape over the left shoulder. The part of the sari that drapes over the shoulder is called a *pallav* and can be worn in various ways: to cover your head or wrapped fully around both shoulders in a shawl style, or left hanging over the left shoulder. The sari is not a difficult garment to wear – after all, in India women do all their daily household chores in them – and there are no size restrictions; it takes the shape of the body and generally slims you down.'

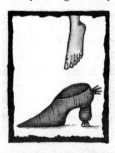

My daughter, aged fifteen, has decided that she is a vegetarian. While I support her wishes and have attempted to cook her tasty veggie food (I come from a big meat-eating family and the only vegetably things I cook are strictly to go with meat . . . but I don't want you to think I am a bad mother!), now she has decided that she won't wear leather. Which poses a problem as far as shoes, belts, etc. are concerned. Please, please, can you help me before I kill her? – *Despairingly yours, South West England*
Oh dear. Let me give you some useful addresses and things so that you can keep her happy and you stay out of jail – jails are such

awful places. Luxury Without Leather make belts out of quality synthetic materials and they look rather nice (call them on 01494 539136 for a brochure). Ethical Wares make outdoor and leisure footwear and clothing without using leather (call 01929 480360 for a colour catalogue) and they have a shop in Brighton (same number). Vegetarian Shoes, also in Brighton (01273 691913), make shoes (surprise!). See, no need to shed blood.

I feel this may be too dull a question for your splendidly frilly column but here goes . . . Is there a way of checking that the clothes I buy are not made by some poor child (or adult) in horrendous conditions? I used to be glad of a bargain but now I'm aware that someone is probably paying the price. Are even M&S really in the clear? I do hope that Traidcraft isn't the only answer! – *Kathryn Rignall, Cheshire*

Nothing is too dull, especially when it is as important an issue as this. The answer, in short, is to ask. One can't really expect the poor old shop assistant to be up on this, but if you shop somewhere regularly you can write to them. This will be good for two reasons: it will give you an answer and it will make them think. I asked M&S what their policy was and they said this: 'Marks & Spencer sources over seventy per cent of its merchandise from the UK, almost £5.4 billion of British-made goods. Of the remaining thirty per cent the major source is Western Europe. A small proportion comes from developing countries. When sourcing overseas, it is our practice to use existing UK suppliers to manage the process. Their long-standing relationship with Marks & Spencer means that they are well aware of the code of conduct we require relating to factory standards, merchandise quality, sound human relations and high environmental standards. In addition, we have a team of technologists who spend a significant proportion of their time visiting factories both in the UK and overseas. A large part of their role is to check that the standards in these factories are being maintained to high levels. We treat, and always have treated, these issues very seriously and they are under regular review.' The Office of Fair Trade in London knew of no way of advising consumers on this subject, ditto your local council trading standards offices. Traidcraft, however, were extremely helpful. They are currently involved in an initiative called the 'Labour Behind the Label' campaign, which aims to raise consumer awareness about this issue (call 0161 247 1760 for more info). Another useful contact is the Oxfam information team on 01865 313600; they are involved in the UK version of an international 'clean clothes' campaign. Hope this helps and thanks to Imogen for all the sterling work she did for me while I soaked my poor swollen feet in a bucket. You may also want to read *No Sweat Fashion, Free Trade, and the Rights of Garment Workers*, edited by Andrew Ross and published by Verso, £14.00.

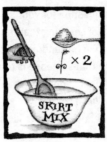

A decade ago I bought the perfect dress. I could still wear it if I hadn't washed it, since when the 'floating' full skirt of voile sticks to the built-in lining when I walk. Is there some preparation I could stick it in?
– A. S. Crocker (Mrs), Bath

This letter caused hugely conflicting advice. You should use fabric conditioner said some; no you shouldn't, said others. Mrs Dobbin from Cheshire wrote in to recommend a Mr H. Berger, Dry Cleaners, Station Road, Cheadle Hulme, Cheshire, who is mysteriously able to reclaim dresses of two materials which have been washed in the wrong substances. Or, Mrs Dobbin suggested, try Woolite in cold water, then the voile skirt can be rinsed out and lightly starched while the underslip can be rinsed in warm water, wrung out, then dipped in a solution of warm water, two tablespoons of glycerine and two of gum arabic stirred together in a plastic bowl, then wring and peg out. Finally, try Go-Stat anti-static spray, which prevents materials from sticking to one another. The product is distributed by Coats Leisure Crafts Group and is available from John Lewis for £2.55.

As a Muslim male I am not allowed to wear silk. This causes me a considerable amount of distress when I have to buy ties. The only place where I currently go is Liberty, who do a range of cotton ties. The problem here is that they only seem to do flowery ones. I try to avoid most high street shops for ties as I'm not keen on being on the tube with several people

wearing the same tie as me. Also most of the polyester ties I seem to find in the high street are of dubious quality/finish. Can you help? Do you know of anybody who would make bespoke ties maybe (at a reasonable price, of course)? – *Saboor Sandhu, London, via e-mail*

I didn't know that Muslim males couldn't wear silk but, in a bit of e-mail exchange, Saboor explained: 'Muslim males are not allowed to wear silk – and also for that matter gold – as they are considered to be the wares of women. The prophet Mohammed was never known to have worn silk garments and advised men not to wear silk.' Fancy, I do love learning new things. OK, Maurice Sedwell, 19 Savile Row, London WIX IAE, tel: 0171 734 0824, has an enormous range of cotton fabrics from which they will happily make bespoke ties for around £50 (it takes two weeks). Paul Smith, 40 Floral Street, London WC2E 9DG, tel: 0171 836 7828, have 100 per cent cotton ties from £35. None of them are silk or of dubious quality, and nor should you meet too many people wearing them. Although after this is printed, who knows . . .

I remember my grandmother talking about using *ash* to clean clothes many years ago. I never thought to ask her how it worked. Do you know? – *Hannah Canvers, London*

I too have heard of this; my mother sometimes talks about this way of doing the laundry. It does sound odd, doesn't it? But basically, the way it worked was ashes were collected (white ashes, not the dirty sooty ones), mixed with water and poured over clothes that had been piled up in big sinks; this was repeated as many times as necessary. The ashy-water mixture is known as lye and the reason it worked was lye is alkaline, which is meant to remove grease, so as it soaked through, the clothes would get clean. Thank goodness AEG came along, eh? (Incidentally, I got this info from a fantastic little book called *Care of Clothes*, published by the National Trust, £4.99. You can buy it at any NT shoppe and it is fascinatingly full of olde worlde stuff like this, and fair does me out of a job.)

I recently purchased a pair of trousers that have 'modal' as part of the ingredients. What is this? I have to say I think it is rather perspiration inducing. Maybe this is why I cannot seem to find a nice girl to fall in love with. I am getting bored with one-night stands. – *Ian, Walthamstow*

First off, Ian, your sartorial enquiry: modal is the generic name for

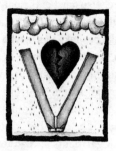

regenerated cellulose fibres, obtained by processes giving a high tenacity and a high wet modulous (all my own words, I swear, Miss). Modal has a high wet strength, which must be useful if you find it makes you sweat (although it should be fairly hydrophilic, maybe it's the other fibres it's mixed with that make you perspire?). Modal has been around for about twenty years. As for the rest of your letter, which I had to edit due to its length, ahem, well then. Sleeping with girls because 'you think it's rude not to' is no way to start a romance, is it? And maybe they are nice girls but you don't give yourself the chance to find out. I have no moral quarrel with one-night lays but for romance one needs to build tension. When I met my husband we circled each other for about two years (I had seen pigeons do it) and by the time we got to hold hands, never mind anything else, I practically fainted. Obviously I'm not saying you should take that long but, really, you can't blame modal for having to drop your trousers quite so soon. Switch to cotton and keep them up.

While in Sydney recently, I tried on a suit made of tensil (apologies for the spelling but until then I hadn't heard of the fabric). Unfortunately, it was the wrong size, so I thought I would look out for something when I got home. Do you know of any stockists in the Bath area? In the places where I've enquired, their ignorance matched mine, and although I have read an article about how it was discovered by the Courtaulds people in Grimsby in the 1980s, the marketplace hardly seems flooded with the product. Thanks for your help. – *Richard Barley, Bath*

Without wishing to sound like a schoolteacher, it's spelt Tencel, it is a fibre not a fabric, and its generic name (in the same way that Lycra's generic name is elastane and Tactel's is nylon) is lyocell. A fibre is, in basic terms, the *stuff* that a *fabric* is made of, i.e., velvet (a fabric) can be made from silk and rayon *fibres*. When Tencel was invented, it was the first new fibre for thirty years and established this new classification (lyocell). It is, indeed, a wonderful fibre, with a good, meaty handle, a bit like a silk fuji or a silk broadsheet. Helen Storey was one of the first to use it in jeans. Now then, on to Tencel's PR people, who were a little reluctant to give info on Tencel, saying that they thought this column was rather 'silly'. Let me explain: it's witty. Rather different from silly – though I do admit that if you've never been called witty, the word 'silly' might be more familiar to you. But the research is anything BUT silly. Stupid girl.

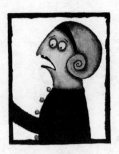

can i? should i?
sometimes

*reassurance for the confused: how to wear
things, when to wear them . . . sartorial
correctness if such a thing exists*

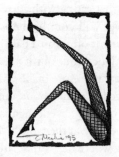

Can I wear fishnets or are they too tarty? – *Helen Jagger, Kensington*

Well, like so many things, it depends on how you wear them. Black fishnets with unintentional holes in them, with red tights underneath and high-heeled red shoes, will look suspect, so don't be surprised if you inspire slow-moving traffic. But yes, fishnets do have a tarty image, which is a shame because they can be fun, they last well, and because they have this hooker association, men can't help staring at your legs (which is nice only if that sort of thing is important to you). Anyway, looking tarty can be a laugh sometimes. But let's suppose that's not what you want. OK, nearly every hosiery company does fishnets of one sort or another, but for a real class pair go to Fogal at 36 New Bond Street, London W1X 9HD, tel: 0171 493 0900. They do beautiful fishnets, from a really fine mesh to a thicker one. There was an ultra-stylish woman in their shop when I went to check them out. She was wearing cream fishnets and they looked divine. She was on her biannual trip to stock up and she looked so good in hers (I have to say I had never thought of wearing cream fishnets) that I felt inspired. Prices are £19 for the wide fishnets and £31 for the very fine ones, sizes S, M and L, and colours include red, black and cream.

I am going to a wedding in August (who isn't?) and wearing a hat for the first time ever! Does one keep one's hat on during the meal? I presume I shall have to discard it by the time I get to the dance floor. I wouldn't normally bother busy people like you with my limited knowledge of fashion protocol, but I can't find the answer to my question in any etiquette books.
– *Barbara King, Lancashire*

Well, I'm not going to a wedding in August, regrettably, as I always find them a great deal of fun. In matters of fashion protocol, I am not much good, since I believe that as long as you don't offend any-one and carry it off with aplomb you should do what you want. My thoughts, however, are that eating with a hat is rather superfluous, especially if the hat is big. Will your hat be easy to take on and off? By that I mean will taking it off mean a half-hour trip to the ladies' to rearrange your hair? Does your outfit *need* the hat and does the removal of your headgear therefore make your outfit 'too simple'? These are things you need to think about, but not for too long. I don't think I have ever been to a wedding that involved hats, and certainly don't remember any at the table. (My best friend, Lily, once went to a wedding where her Aunt Catherine kept her hat on and secreted all manner of antipasto under it, to take home to give to her cats – she was that sort of woman – but I doubt you will be doing that.) Men remove their top hats (if they are wearing them) at the table, and I think it only fair, in the interests of equality, that women do the same. I would perhaps keep the hat on when you first sit down, if toasts and whatnot are performed at the beginning of the meal, and then take it off for eating. But ultimately, do what feels comfortable and sod protocol.

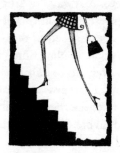

Is it OK to wear a G-string with a short skirt? – *Sally Tyvek, Sidcup*
There was once a girl of my acquaintance who wore thong panties constantly. She also had a penchant for miniskirts, and usually combined the two very well. She was careful, you know, bending over and climbing up stairs (maintaining a straight back, she informed me, was the key to a successful discreet ascent). Then, one horrible day, she brought a rucksack to work with her when rucksacks were just becoming fashionable (this girl was at the cutting edge of fashion). She hitched it on to her back, not noticing, dear reader, that the rucksack had hitched up her short skirt with it. She happily walked to work thinking she must look very good indeed today: she could hear wolf whistles behind her and builders

swung off scaffolding shouting urgent things at her. It was only when she got to work and stood in the mirrored-wall lift that she realized her bottom was on general display. She was never the same after that. Other than avoiding rucksacks, there is no reason why you shouldn't wear G-strings under a short skirt. Personally I can't see why you can't wear anything you want under a short skirt, including nothing at all if the fancy takes you (provided you are careful, so as not to get arrested for indecency). And be extra careful going up escalators. If you see a gaggle of men loitering at the bottom with a zoom-lens camera, you can bet it's not the novelty-painted ceiling they're snapping.

Is it OK to wear navy with black? And what about blue with green?
– Veronica Walsh, Lewisham
Yes, yes.

How high should heels be for work? – *Tessa Malcolm, St Ives*
What sort of work? Generally, as long as you can walk in them then they are OK. If you are a prozzie, then I guess they can be as high as you like as you will spend most of your time lying down, or against a wall. A rule of thumb is: if the ball of your foot still touches the floor, then you're OK. If not, we're talking fetish.

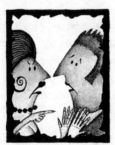

My husband insists on wearing his polo shirts done right up to the neck. I think it looks wrong and keep undoing the top button. Short of cutting all the top buttons off and pretending they got lost in the washing machine, what can I do? – *Helen Belgo, Jersey*
There is no right or wrong way of wearing a polo shirt, but I agree doing it right up to the top looks a bit 'uptight'. I think cutting the buttons off is a bit devious – how would you like it if he did a similar thing to your clothes? Flattery is the best solution here. Saying things like, 'God, I love the way Gary Oldman/Leonardo

DiCaprio /Robert Carlyle wears his shirt with one button undone like that, showing just a bit of chest, it's sooo sexy,' to a girlfriend over the phone, making sure he overhears, will work wonders. But be subtle, men aren't *that* stupid.

I saw a Vivienne Westwood suit in her shop which is quite divine but costs £541 (it is a fitted wool jacket with three buttons and has a matching pencil skirt). I have the money to buy it (just) and I think it is fairly classic, but my mother says Vivienne Westwood is 'wacky'. She wants me to spend the money on a suit from Jigsaw or Marks & Spencer, which she says will stand the test of time. Should I buy the VW suit or listen to my mother?
– *Wendy Harris, Strand on the Green*

Jigsaw and M&S do excellent suits, but there is no way they can compare with one from Vivienne Westwood. The woman is a genius and her suits are classic, sexy, superbly made and cut, and an investment. Some of them are more extreme than others, granted, but choose well (and the one you describe sounds perfect, not too 'wacky' at all). There are loads of boring suits on the market – stand out and fork out. And if you are ever in doubt again, follow this catch-all maxim that I have invented to help me through life: 'Buy it, do it, eat it.' It answers just about every question life can throw at you.

I have a black sleeveless dress. Sometimes my bra (black) strap peeks out from under my dress. I think it looks quite sweet, but my friend recently told me it looks tarty. What do you think?
– *Esther Connell-Turner, Taunton*

I agree with you that a bit of bra strap showing can look nice. After all, it is nothing to be ashamed of. In places like Spain and Italy, women frequently have bra straps showing. Far better to be confident with a bit of peek-a-boo strap than to be constantly fiddling to tuck it in. What sort of friend tells you that you look tarty with so little provocation? I'll bet she has washerwoman's upper arms and so never dares to show hers. Next time your friend comments on your bra strap, mention that you have some sheets that need washing.

I like wearing fairly see-through blouses and am careful to wear 'matching' bras: i.e., black for black, cream for cream, etc. Most of these shirts have shoulder pads which you can see. Someone at work said this was highly tacky. Is it? – *Wanda, Shropshire*

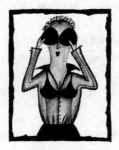

I'd say. Although I am mellowing in my old age and think people should essentially wear what they wish to, I can't help thinking that a see-through blouse is the woman's equivalent of a red sport's car. And why were you wearing such a thing at work? Anyway, you have asked me one thing and I must stick to the point. Shoulder pads are suspect at the best of times (although they keep trying to make a comeback, thanks mostly to Alexander McQueen), so visible shoulder pads become very suspect things indeed. If you must wear blouses that show your bra, please take the shoulder pads out. If necessary, wear them as blinkers.

There is this girl at work who keeps telling me that my skirts are too short. I am twenty-one, have nice legs (I think) and wear opaque tights and low shoes with them. I am very careful when I bend down. She says short skirts are very 1980s and now women don't have to show their legs, but I like wearing short skirts and don't think I'll be able to wear them when I'm older. What do you think? – *Simone, Portsmouth*

Oh yes, and what does she look like? Like a sumo wrestler, I'll bet. Women can be their own worst enemy. I can't stand this female bitchy backhandedness. You sound sensible, sexy and nice. Of course you can wear short skirts. Women have a choice now and you've made yours. Next time sumo makes a comment, smile and say, 'Goodness, you look nice today. Where's that lovely jumper/skirt/tent from?' This'll fox her. As one of the characters in *Absolutely Fabulous* once said, 'In with anger, out with love.'

I am sixty and fairly pale. I am unsure what colours to wear for my top half, as I seem to look so washed out these days. I have some great 'bargains' – blouses and tops that I have bought over the years in pale peach, cream, etc. Should I give them to charity or brazen it out? My sister-in-law recently told me they 'did nothing for me' and whereas once I wore them every so

often, now I feel too nervous to. Can I wear paler colours at my age?
– *Mrs Bishop, Bristol*

What is going on with all this bitchiness! All you need to do is add a brightly coloured scarf and that will bring colour to your face and allow you to wear what you damn well please. And remember that charity begins at home, so keep the blouses and give your sister-in-law to charity.

I have one quick question for you. I know you have a huge waiting list, but please, please try to fit this in. I saw a Jil Sander suit which is a shade over £1,000 (I can't write the exact figure in, I'm too embarrassed). I'm not rich but I can just afford it. I am in a total quandary as to whether to buy it. I'm usually decisive but I CAN'T DECIDE WHAT TO DO. All my friends say I am mad to spend so much on a suit. Should I buy it? – *Rebecca, Kent*

Oh, Rebecca. You want me to give you permission, don't you? You want me to say, 'It's OK, it's investment dressing.' Stop getting yourself into such a flap. Buy the suit. Jil Sander is a supremely classic designer and you will no doubt wear it loads. It will not go out of fashion and as long as you're not going to starve if you spend the money on this suit, then OF COURSE YOU SHOULD BUY IT, YOU SILLY GIRL. Anyway, wearing a Jil Sander suit will no doubt elicit all sorts of dinner-date invites, so you won't go hungry. Your friends are obviously jealous. So start practising writing the amount on your chequebook. P.S. Don't even consider having children if the purchase of an item of clothing reduces you to a gibbering, indecisive wreck.

How can I dress so that people think I am fashionable and metropolitan?
– *P.W., Loughton*

Dear P.W., why would you want to? You dress how you damn well please and heed this great saying by, I believe, the preacher James DeWeerd: 'It is better to die on the horeb of isolation knowing you've been true to yourself than to rot away in the mephitic alleys of the commonplace.' There is a ridiculous pressure these days to conform to fashion, but remember that what is fashionable and metropolitan today will be yesterday's news tomorrow.

My mum has just 'inherited' a Burberry raincoat from my grandad. She thinks it quite stylish and it fits her well. It has padded shoulders, is loose fitting and comes to just below the knee. The problem is that it's that material that changes colour in the light – green to purple to orange. I think it is

quite naff. What do you think? Before she makes serious fools of us all.
– *Georgie Cooke (aged fourteen), Shropshire*

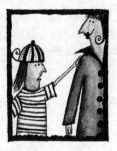

I have never heard of a Burberry raincoat that does such a thing. Some have a subtle sheen to them (I can only *assume* you're exaggerating) but nothing as trippy as what you describe. Well, Georgie, let me tell you a little bit about Burberry trench-coats. Thomas Burberry created gabardine in the 1870s and this is the fabric that most Burberrys are still made from. Gabardine is very hard-wearing, keeps the rain out, doesn't crease and is a joy to wear. Lots of debonair young men wore gabardine – Amundsen, Scott and Shackleton wore it to the South Pole. As did Alcock and Brown when they became the first men to fly the Atlantic in 1919; and A. E. Clouston, who, with Mrs Betsy Kirby-Green, made the fastest time to Cape Town from London in 1937 (six hours and forty-five minutes). Burberry trench-coats were officially sanctioned by the War Office and the Admiralty and were worn by half a million officers in the Great War (1914–18) – hence the 'trench-coat' name. The 'D' rings were for attaching grenades to the front and a sword at the back. Kitchener died in his Burberry trench-coat. After the war, these brave young men brought their trenches home and they became part of everyday life after that. Peter Sellers wore one in *The Pink Panther Strikes Again* and loved it so much that he kept two, just in case. So you see what a romantic history (although there is nothing romantic about war) Burberry's trench-coats have? Look at your mother with pride; there is nothing naff about her heirloom, and remember it might be yours one day. They last quite a while.

Is it ever acceptable to wear tights with open-toed sandals? Of course I mean very sheer, natural tights. Are they OK, or does that webbing-effect round the toes look a bit strange? – *Hester, Battersea*

No, it's not, and yes, it does. Acknowledge the seasons with your little feet, Hester, and let them go naked when the sun shines.

Should I wear V-neck and round-neck jumpers with different outfits (for example, with a tie), and if so, how? Or is one type intrinsically more stylish than the other? – *Paul Miller, Nottingham*
There really doesn't seem any point in wearing a round neck with a shirt and tie. More stylish by far to wear one with a grandad-collar shirt (and no tie). Neither is particularly stylish – jumpers tend to be casual and don't mix well with shirt and tie, but at a pinch a V-neck is better. A more stylish option is to wear a plain knitted waistcoat with your shirt and tie. Try Paul Smith, 40 Floral Street, London WC2E 9DG, tel: 0171 836 7828, who often do them.

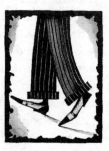

I like to wear slip-on shoes with my formal suits but my girlfriend says they make me look like a pimp. Who's right? – *Tony Roston, Bedford*
It depends – if the suit is funky, then slip-on shoes (with stacked heel) may look good, but you'll still look like a pimp. If the suit is more conformist, then only polished brogues or Oxford lace-ups will do.

If I buy a Moschino bikini costing £100, is it all right to wear the knickers inside out so that the label shows? – *A. MacDonald (Mrs), Dorset*
Oh dear, no. People will think you have gone quite mad if you wander round the beach with your gusset on show. Surely the stupendous cut of the Moschino bikini will indicate it is a designer number and not something you picked off the floor in some cheap store's changing rooms.

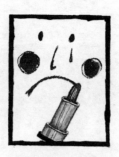

long-lost loves
sniff no more
*a scent, label or particular jumper you loved
and can't find any more is tracked down*

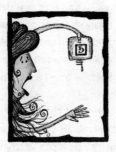

For years I was a fan of the products of Cosmetics to Go. I understand that they went bankrupt and I was overjoyed when they reappeared under the new name Lush. However, the one product that I really wanted had disappeared – that sublime perfume, Ginger, to which I am addicted. The shop assistant told me that there was some kind of patent row between the new Lush and the creator of Ginger, and that the perfume would never be available again. Is this true? Is there any way I can get hold of Ginger again? It is the nicest scent I have ever bought. Please tell me how I can prevail upon these short-sighted perfume people to bring me back my Ginger.
– *Catherine Richards, Bethnal Green, London*

Right, then, let's clear some stuff up. Cosmetics to Go were owned by a company called Constantine & Weir until May 1994, when CTG were sold to a company called Fountainhall Marketing UK Ltd. I spoke to a lovely lass at Cosmetics to Go called Marcia, so you see they still exist, they still produce a catalogue and they still make Ginger! Yippee! Lush is an entirely different company. I am unsure which shop assistant you spoke to – Cosmetics to Go no longer have a shop; they operate entirely by mail order – but she was clearly talking nonsense. CTG make a Ginger range, from their famous bath bombs, called Ginger Snaps, £3.10 for two, to the famous Ginger perfume, £14.50. They also do soap and a bath oil. There is even a Ginger FM (for men). I hope you and your Ginger will be reunited soon. Call Cosmetics to Go on 01202 621966 for a catalogue. (Anyone who hasn't tried their stuff really should, it's original and fun and makes you feel like a kid again, as their products come to you all nestled in what look like recycled shredded paper and they quite often used to put in little pressies, like sticks of rock, for you to hunt out.)

The only jeans that I have ever been comfortable in are Levi's 901's. Now, goodness knows why, they have been discontinued and replaced with

some awful design with no waist and legs that don't taper (541 or something). I have been into as many shops as possible searching for any remaining pairs and have tried to find out why they have disappeared – I presume I must have been the only person who bought them. Yesterday my last blue pair developed a hole, so now I am desperate. What shall I do?
– *Naomi, London*

The Levi's PR people confirmed that Levi's 901's have been discontinued. They first appeared in 1986 and were sold exclusively in the UK. They advise that the best bet is to go to Personal Pair at the Levi's flagship store, 174 Regent Street, London WIR 5DE, tel: 0171 439 2028, where you are measured and the jeans are customized to suit your shape and taste. You normally have to wait three weeks for the jeans. This will probably be the nearest you get to anything like 901's. They will be more comfortable; the only downside is that they are, of course, more expensive: approx. £65.

I wrote to you last year and you never replied so I thought I'd try again. I want slip-on plimsoles, like you used to wear at school. They're great for summer. Please, please, find some for me. I'll be your best friend for ever.
– *Imogen, Cirencester*

'Be my bessie, eh?' And let me use all your felt-tip pens? Thank you but no thank you, I have a best friend already and splendid she is too. I remember you from last year – I'm sorry I didn't reply, I wish I could to everyone but I can't. So then, you persistent girlie. I know what you mean. Racing Green (0345 331177) do some really pretty ones for £15 in various colours, called the Mary Anne. They also do the Nautical plimsole in red or navy (gusset is striped), £17, both in sizes 36–42. So plod off now and stop stalking me.

I am looking for a replacement for a fourteen-year-old pair of Dunlop Green Flash tennis pumps (or daps, depending on which bit of the UK you went to school in). They have kept my feet warm, dry and comfortable in last year's northern Italian snow, this year's Harwich snow (albeit with furry insoles), as well as in the filthy heat of Athens, London and Rome. I am prepared to brave the derision of the youths who sell trainers in sports shops, but only if I can get these Green Flash things (or – even better – the Red Flash, which were The Thing at school in the 1960s). My Nike-clad son will die if you print this request, but I have told him that only Italians know good shoes when they see them, and I've yet to see an Italian lady in Nikes.
– *Jenny, Bedford*

Well, to spare your son's premature death, I have omitted your surname. And *I* wear Nikes to run in, so although you haven't seen
me, that blows your theory. Now then, your pumps or plimsoles as
I call them. The good news is that you won't have to brave the
derision of any snotty youths as Green Flash are stocked by that
wonderful institution, and my favourite store, Johnny Loulou.
They come in sizes 6–12 (half-sizes aren't stocked but can be
ordered) and cost £15. They don't stock Red Flash and I don't
know anyone who does; I tried all my trainer contacts to no avail.

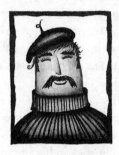

One of my abiding memories of childhood (during the 1950s and 1960s) is
the sight of my father (deceased) – a Polish refugee – wearing a beret (of the
type worn by Frenchmen). I am now forty-one and find that I enjoy things my
father did at that age. I would like a beret but have no idea where I might be
able to buy one. My hopes were raised at the recent Heineken Cup Final
match between my team, Leicester Tigers, and the French team Brive. I
hoped to be able to persuade a Frenchman to part with his beret as an
exchange for my rugby shirt but did not get the opportunity. I noticed that
some berets had a peak (worn at the back) and I thought how elegant they
looked. Please could you let me know where I might be able to buy such a
beret. I live in Leicester but work in central London. – *Zdzislaw Matusiewicz*
What a lovely letter. But it made me rather sad that at forty-one
you no longer have your daddy, because daddies are important
things. A traditional French beret, also called a Basque beret, is different from the usual ones because it has a leather band around the
crown. I have just returned from Switzerland, where I bought
myself a fabulous Swiss Army knife (after having wanted one for
ever – my husband refused to buy me one) and I did look out for
one there for you. However, the Hat Shop do them! Yippee. They
come in eight different sizes and cost £17.75; contact them at 14
Lamb Street, Spitalfields, London E1 6EA, tel: 0171 247 1120 (they

do a catalogue as well and it's in there). Be happy – now you won't have to swap any part of your wardrobe to get one.

My problem is finding a replacement lipstick. My mother and her generation – I am sixty – used to use a wonderful orange-looking Tangee lipstick (natural) available from Woolworth all through the war years, 1939–45. A whole generation of women used this Tangee natural lipstick. It went out of production in the 1960s, but my mother had collected boxes of lipstick from Britain and the USA which I have been using until now and I am down to my last one! The orange shade takes on a pinky hue when applied to the lips and is very long-lasting, moisturizes the lips and is an excellent product. I have tried other lipsticks but cannot find anything to replace it. Ask anyone aged sixty-plus if their mothers used the lipstick and they will say, 'Oh yes, it was wonderful!' I have tried in vain to find a replacement. Can you please help?
– Angeline Levy, Aberdeen

An orange lipstick that takes on a pinky hue? It sounds well spooky to me. Da na na na, da na na na. I don't know where to begin with this one. My mother's over sixty, bless her, but she doesn't look it, and she has never used a lipstick in her life so she was no good helping with this. But if this is as widespread a phenomenon as you say, then I should hope to be inundated with helpful women writing in to tell me what they've replaced it with. Come on, you old birds, there's a snog with Shane Ritchie in it for you.

And it was a phenomenon, here are some answers from readers:

I'm just reading Elizabeth Jane Howard's *The Light Years* and in Part One there is a description of Louise's possessions – including her 'precious Tangee lipstick that looked bright orange but came out pink on the mouth'.
– Pam Dye, Chiddingly, East Sussex

Thank you for this cultural reference. More of this and I'll be on the arts pages! Yes, please.

I'll pass on the Shane Ritchie snog, thanks, but there is a lipstick made by Ultra Glow of Colchester that comes close to Tangee natural: Magic Lips comes in loads of colours, all of which not only take on more traditional colours when applied but also last much longer and better than other widely advertised 'long-lasting' brand lipsticks. Another excellent lipstain is made by Colorsport and comes in eight colours, from pink to red through bronze. Both of these products can be found in independent chemist shops rather than stores or chain chemists. They retail at about £3.95.
– Anna Farlow, London

Thanks. Barbara Donovan from Cardiff also suggested Magic Lips, saying it's 'green in the tube and pink on the lips'.

I am seventy and Tangee lipstick was the first lipstick I used in my teens during the war. I don't think there was much choice then. I still like a pinky lipstick and use Avon Tender Pink. – *Mrs Perrin, Great Missenden, Bucks*

And a Mrs Feuchtwanger rang me and told me that it was 'one's first lipstick when one was a teenager and it got past headmistresses and parents'. Oh, I feel a film coming on . . . Finally, my suggestion for what it's worth, as I am famous for eating off my lipgloss . . . Clinique's Glosswear with Brush SPF8, which must be the most unromantic name for a lipgloss ever. It's subtle and great for people like me who are frightened of lipstick, costs £8 and comes in lots of nice colours (call 0171 409 6951 if you can't find a stockist near you).

I use just such a lipstick; and a green one which goes deep pink! (There is also a yellow one that turns coral and a pale blue one that turns pale lilac pink.) They change according to the alkali content of your lips, stay on most of the day and cost £1 at the South Molton Drug Store in South Molton Street, London w1. This is the only place I can find that stocks them, but there have to be others. If Mrs Levy can't get them herself, give her my address. – *Judy Nicholls, Kent*

Bless you, Judy. Mrs Levy, my love, if you're still having trouble finding them, get back in touch and I shall go down to the SMS Pharmacy myself and get you some! If anyone is interested, their number is 0171 493 4156.

Do you know the address of the Mary Quant Cosmetics mail-order service. I'd like to replace a lipstick I bought several years ago.
– *Nina Ashby, Aberdeen*

You can place your order or ask for a catalogue by calling 0171 581 1811.

On my quest for the perfect jeans, I happened, a couple of years ago, to find a pair of Levi's 620's. These are the perfect cut and ever since I have been searching for another pair. (Mine are starting to 'go' – sob, sob!) I've been told that they were discontinued years ago, hence I bought mine from a charity shop. I was wondering if perhaps Levi's have a warehouse or something that carries their old lines? Hope against hope, I bet! Now you know my story, could you do a bit of detective work for me, as I wouldn't know where to start! Can you save me from rummaging for evermore for my

620's so I can have time looking for other super-trendy super-cheap stuff
from Scope and Oxfam? Do your stuff, Annie!
– *Kerry Mason, Crawley, West Sussex*

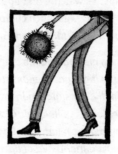

Levi's don't have a warehouse with all their old lines. Would that
they did, because I get hundreds of requests from people searching
out long-loved, now lost, Levi's [there's one a bit further back in this
very chapter]. Your beloved 620's were around in this country about
eight or nine years ago. They were a very tight fit, with an orange
tab, but were phased out and replaced by 611's, which were phased
out quite recently. Today, the closest you will find to them are the
505 red tab or the 595 red tab. These are available at Original Levi's
Stores nationwide. The one in Brighton is at 168 Weston Road and
the general enquiries number for Levi's stockists is 01604 790436. I
also contacted vintage clothes store 1920s–1970s Crazy Clothes
Connection, 134 Lancaster Road, London W11 1QU, tel: 0171 221
3989, who said they do get them in occasionally but not regularly
and when they do they start at £125 (for a pair of jeans, goodness!).
If you're really fond of them, it is worth calling into Crazy Clothes
every now and again and checking. Vintage jeans shop Rokit, 225
Camden High Street, London NW1 7BU, tel: 0171 267 3046, have a
massive selection of second-hand Levi's and they might be worth a
try, but they don't get them in regularly.

**Please help. I'm desperate to get a new pair of Brothel Creepers, the kind
with the 2" sole. My only pair are falling apart after nearly two years, but I'm
persevering because I can't find them anywhere. Something sturdy, leather,
with thick soles that won't fall apart when I go out disco-dancing. Thank
you. P. S. I'd prefer laces and I take a size 4. –** *Sarah Dempsey, Glasgow*
Hello, Sarah. Ad Hoc, 153 King's Road, London SW3 5TX, tel: 0171
376 1121 and 28 Kensington Church Street, London W8 4EP, tel:
0171 938 1664 have exactly what you want, black leather brothel

creepers which come in sizes 3–12, from £50. So either go visit if you're ever here or ring them and tell them exactly what you want; you pay by credit card and they post them to you (or you can send a cheque). Or visit the Shelly's in Glasgow; they do some suitable things (I'm not being purposely woolly here, just that it changes lots). Ring them on 0181 450 0066; they also do mail order. When they do them, they come in sizes 4–8 and cost around the £50 mark.

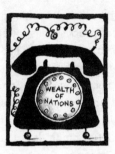

Several times over the past year or so you have mentioned one of my favourite sources of clothes, Wealth of Nations, in your 'Dear Annie' column. I have been looking forward to seeing their new catalogue. So much so that I phoned them to find out when it would arrive. I tried their old number and got a BT-ish announcement, referring me on to another number. I tried the second number, which has a constant 'busy now' announcement/message and which does not respond, ever. Has Wealth of Nations gone out of business? Heaven forbid, have I missed their change of address details/am I *persona non grata*/have they all been kidnapped in Kashmir or shanghaied in China or incarcerated in India? Can you help please?
– Susan, Cambridge

For a while back there I was flummoxed too. I tried calling every number I had for them. I tried writing to them, only to have the letter come back, Elvis fashion, marked 'Return to Sender'. Let me try to explain: Wealth of Nations, the name and mailing lists, were purchased in July 1997 (they were in receivership at the time) by the company which now runs it, Judy French, who have been established for several years as a ladieswear manufacturer. There are some favourites from previous collections included and it's still the same idea – clothes from around the world – but the clothes are not as 'ethnic' as before. The new owners aren't liable for any outstanding debts (they have no connection with the original company whatsoever). But as an act of goodwill, they did send out letters of apology and offered 50 per cent discounts off their first orders to customers who hadn't received refunds for garments returned to the original WON (but orders had to be placed before a certain date, which has now passed). I hope that explains things. It's rum luck when this sort of thing happens, but I'm pleased to see the WON brochure has been relaunched. Call 01689 816 600 for a catalogue or orders. It definitely works!

Please help and please ignore the twee writing paper, it was all that was available. My two favourite lipstick shades – Acajou and Amarante – both made by Bourjois, have been discontinued. I had heard that Bourjois is a sort of test range for a more expensive cosmetics company. Is this true and if so, who is it, and more importantly, do they now do shades that are the equivalents of my favourites? Thank you very much.
– Louise Holmes, Stockport

Heresy, Bourjois is not a test range! It is a fabulous range in its own right. Bourjois has been going for 133 years. It began supplying make-up for theatre stars in France in the late nineteenth century, and can boast stars like Sandra Bernhardt. I think the confusion about Bourjois, and what has given rise to a few 'urban myths', is that it is a sister brand to Chanel. The colours you seek were discontinued last year but there are similar shades in the new lipstick range called Eclat de Rire. The shade closest to Acajou is Cannelle (number 34). The shade closest to Amarante is Garance (number 33). They are available at Boots and Superdrug, costing £5.45 each. There is a free stockist enquiry number: 0800 269836. I hope the shades find favour with you.

Once upon a time you could buy sensuous men's underwear and night wear from a mail-order firm called Après Noir. They don't appear to exist any more. I'm not a TV, I don't want women's clothes, just slinky nylon (not satin), that makes me feel sexy. – Fred, Northumberland

I care not the hole in a doughnut (mmm . . . now that's a thought) if you are a TV or not, Fred. You don't need to explain to me, you sauce . . . You can obtain Après Noir from Body Aware, 98 Meadows Works, Trowbridge, Wiltshire, BA14 8BR, tel: 01225 774164. There is also a website: www.bodyaware.com; e-mail address: services@bdyaware.demon.co.uk.

My husband's favourite casual evening wear is a fine merino wool sweater with long sleeves, collar and three-button opening at the neck (with

trousers, of course!). In the past our local family-run menswear shop has ordered them for him from John Smedley, but we were told last week that this firm no longer makes a small-size sweater, which is what my husband has always had (he is 37"). It has always been difficult to buy men's sweaters in size Small, so this news is quite a blow. As you can see, we live quite a distance from a major shopping centre, though this is not normally a problem, so any help you can give will be very much appreciated.

– *Marjorie Richardson, Truro, Cornwall*

As I thought, this is simply not true. John Smedley still make Small, but not many shops buy it. It makes me so ANGRY when shops say, 'The manufacturers don't make them any more,' when what they mean is they don't sell them. Call the lovely John Smedley menswear enquiry line on 0171 734 1519; they can tell you who does sell the sweaters near you and they can even possibly post them out to you. The style you mention is still made and costs £65. Or go back to your old stockist and put them right!

A good friend's ex divorced him because he, among other things, would not throw out his thirty-year-old, well-worn, army-issue string vest. I am coming under pressure over my forty-year-old, navy-issue seaman's jersey. But I cannot find anything like it anywhere. It is not the shape, a standard no-frills T with a crew neck, or the colour, navy, but what it is made out of. It is a fine wool yarn which knits up at about ten rows to the inch. This makes it a garment which is cool yet warm, still stretchy (it is close-fitting) and throws off moisture like a raincoat. A thread from the tattered cuff is enclosed. Please help me. I do not know who the winner will be if I have to choose between my wife and my seaman's jersey.

– *Tom Taylor, Highgate, London*

Ooh, Tom, well don't chuck out Mrs T just yet because I don't know if I can get you a replacement jersey to keep you warm. I phoned Silverman Military Clothing, 2 Harford Street, London E1 4PS, tel: 0171 790 0900, for a catalogue. The manager, Malcolm, said he hasn't seen them around for a long time and he can't think of where you might get one. The new navy crew necks he described that they do sounded too thick – they cost from about £20, depending on size. I also tried Laurence Corner, but they had never seen one. They suggested the National Maritime Museum in Greenwich, who couldn't help, and the Imperial War Museum thought the nearest you would find to it for its gauge and water-repellent qualities is an oiled Guernsey. I also spoke to the Defence

Clothing and Textile Agency, who put me on to a lieutenant who knows about these things, apparently, but he was on leave. They also said I should try some ex-bishop who is a knitwear expert, but at this stage my family needed me to cook dinner and I gave up. If anyone out there can help, get in touch please . . .

. . . and people did. Carole Gray, bless you, from Bishop's Stortford e-mailed me to say that she was at a craft fair in Whitby one Saturday and there was a stall selling 'Traditional Fishermen's Ganseys', which were very similar to the usual sort but thinner (she says). The company is called Bob-bins and they sell kits to make them up. Their number is 01947 600585. Fancy that – there Carole is on a Saturday and she thinks of Tom's jumper! . . . Bloody marvellous. And Nurhan contacted me via e-mail to suggest Force 4, a sailing shop in London's Victoria (0171 828 3900). And a sweet-sounding lady from Cambridge called Alice who knits babies' shawls said that she could get the two-ply wool and would knit him one. I put the two in touch but don't know whether Tom's wife was saved.

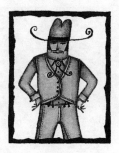

tv
as seen on tv or at the movies
*how to dress like your heroes from
the silver screen*

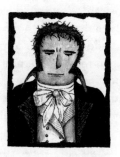

As a *Pride and Prejudice* addict, I was transfixed by the sight of Colin Firth's amazing frothy white shirt collars. I am not sure exactly what they are called (stock, jabot or what?) but I cannot imagine any man would not be improved by a similar garment. Are such things still available and would you have to have a manservant to help you get into it in the morning?
– *Robert Millan, Putney*

Well, a stock collar is like a strip of fabric worn around the collar (like in riding dress or a clerical collar) and a jabot is the spill of lace you would get in Highland dress or the frill on the front of a man's shirt. It is a most romantic style of shirt, conjuring up images of Mr Rochester and, as you say, Darcy types. In fact, when I first met my husband he was wearing a frilly shirt, which, coupled with a bristly attitude, was most attractive. Anyway, these shirts are not easy to get hold of. Angels Fancy Dress, costumiers to the entertainment industry, told me that it is a period shirt from 1810 and the collar is referred to as a Byron collar. There is no official name for it; this is how it was referred to at the time. They do one (i.e., a shirt with this type of collar) which you can hire (and thus you can see how it goes) for £15 + VAT and a deposit of £50 (returnable): contact them at 119 Shaftesbury Avenue, London WC2H 8AD, tel: 0171 836 5678. They do the costumes for various films which you can hire for fancy dress afterwards (currently in, those from *Titanic*, *The Wings of the Dove*, *The Man in the Iron Mask*, *Mrs Brown*, *Amistad*, etc., etc.), so it is well worth a visit anyway. And no, you wouldn't need a manservant to help you into it, unless you are really very cack-handed.

Hello. I've been watching reruns of *The Avengers* and am now lusting after a Victorian-style smoking jacket. Does anyone make them?
– *Robert Ashdown, Dorset*

Thank you for your postcard. You sound like a splendid fellow. I feel I have failed slightly in that I have not found any stockists near you. Favourbrook in London (0171 491 2337) do a few styles that you may like. I realize that they are not near, you but if you call them they can send you a small catalogue which shows you a selection of garments, including two of their smoking jackets. Prices start at £380. Or try Bertie Wooster, 284 Fulham Road, London SW10 9EW, tel: 0171 352 5662. They sell second-hand smoking jackets starting from a slightly cheaper £150. They are in velvet and the oldest is from the 1960s. I hope you do occasionally come to London, as otherwise I shall have been of no help.

My wife and I saw the film _A Month by the Lake_ recently. It is set in the 1930s and in it Edward Fox wears a bathing costume, a one-piece shorts and vest combination with no sleeves. I thought he looked quite marvellous in it and I would like to know where, if possible, I could obtain a similar one. Thank you for your help. – _Robert Freidus, London_
I have about one of these letters a week, for these sorts of gentlemen's old-fashioned bathing suits. The reason they are so difficult to find is that the old ones were made of wool and tended to get a bit moth-eaten. If you want to be really authentic and get a knitted one, it's Angels Fancy Dress (0171 836 5678) to the rescue again, but only if you want to hire one. Otherwise, ring the fantastic Splash Out, who make swimwear made to measure (01903 230861). They can make you one for about £40 upwards. Which is a bloody bargain.

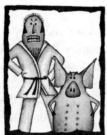

Honey, what I really want is the top that Renton wears at the end _Trainspotting_. It is a clinging turquoise V-neck of the kind that is available from Ted Baker, Nicole Farhi . . . but it is long-sleeved and the shade of blue is cooler than any of the above do. Also I need the belt the men wear in _Much Ado About Nothing_ (fashion summed up in a nutshell). They are

dark brown and chunky with unpretentious buckles – a bit like one of the Timberland ones, but without the maker's name on. Please put me out of my misery. I would very much appreciate any help you could give me (and no, I don't get all my clothes ideas from films). – *Love Tom, Chester*

Look, Tom, we hardly know each other and already you have called me honey and signed off with love. My husband is extremely high-ranking in one of the martial arts disciplines, as well as being a bloody brilliant pig farmer and more than able to play, and sing along with, the guitar – even when drunk. He saw your apricot-coloured *billet-doux* to me and started strumming and singing some James Taylor song, which *always* means he is sulking. Anyway, I have found out for you exactly where that top came from. I went straight to the top – to the costume designer on *Trainspotting*, Rachael Fleming, who was gloriously helpful and told me that the top is by a company called Free (0171 498 1349). I rang Free, who told me that if you ring them they will send you one mail order, as there isn't a stockist near you (the nearest one is Drome in Liverpool). Now then, belts. I have two suggestions here. The first one involves Camden, where there is a stand by the lock that makes belts to order. I can't remember the name and I couldn't get down there to do a recce for you, but you sound like a young lad who can do a bit of footwork (and may I remind you that I have five kids under ten, not much fun on a Saturday in Camden). Second, Frogpool Manor Saddlery (0181 300 0716) can make belts to order. It takes two to three weeks and costs from £18, depending on width and length; colours are limited to black and two types of brown, but it certainly sounds as if they could make you the chunky belt you require. In the meantime, stop watching so many films and get yourself a girlfriend. Honey.

I am a big fan of Jane Austen and the Regency period and would love to get a Regency or Regency-style dress, but have not a clue where to get one. I've tried a few antique shops, but none of them could help. Is there anywhere I could purchase what I want? I'm sure that after the immensely popular dramatization of *Pride and Prejudice* on TV, everyone must be looking for Regency garments! – *Lydia Edwards (age thirteen), Wilmslow, Cheshire*

Mmm, empire-line dresses are rather fab, aren't they? I bought a gorgeous cream one from Top Shop a few years ago and it is my most favourite dress. But this look is rather 'bosomy' and although I don't want to sound like your mum, you shouldn't be showing

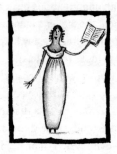

your chest at thirteen, other than to your doctor. But I expect you want an interpretation of this look, don't you? (Incidentally, I see that watching such period dramas has affected you rather more than just sartorially – 'but have not a clue where to get one' is hardly thirteen-year-old speak, is it? Good on you, concentrate on the English and leave boys to their conkers.) Look for empire-line dresses (although the more correct term for this is 'vertical line') in places like Dorothy Perkins, the aforementioned Top Shop and Miss Selfridge and add some Regency touches, such as chopping off your cardigans to just below bust level to wear over a dress [see Paula's problem next], tying a length of ribbon below the bust on a simple shift (you need to run a few stitches over the ribbon) and wearing your hair in curls. If you are handy with a needle, you can get some really great dressmaking patterns from Amazon's Vinegar & Pickling Works Dry Goods (fantastic name, huh?) on tel: 001 319 322 6800, fax: 001 319 322 4003. If it's cheaper for you to write to them for a catalogue/information, their address is 2218 East 11th Street, Davenport, Iowa 52803-3780, USA. They are 'Purveyors of needed items for the 19th Century impression' and are fabulous. They have all sorts of 'patterns from other eras' and have a day dress one that would be ideal for you. Have fun.

I was also very inspired by *Pride and Prejudice*. How can I add subtle Regency touches to my everyday dress without looking like I am in costume? And is it appropriate ever to show that much bosom during the day? – *Paula Murray, London*

Bosoms are a part of a woman's body, so there should be no shame in displaying them, but we all know that we live in a strange world, where breasts are regarded with curiosity and suspicion. Show your tits and you are instantly regarded as a loose woman. Strange, then, that in Jane Austen's day, when people didn't even kiss before marriage, so much flesh was regularly shown. So my sensible advice would be: do not show that much bosom during the day, save it for the evening. As for how to add subtle Regency touches, well, anything empire line will now elicit cries of 'Oh, very Jane Austen' (I know, I've been there). I gave Lydia some cheaper places to go, but as you can afford a bit more the very best place to go to get you started is Ghost (tel: 0171 229 1057), where you can get fabulous dresses for about £100, and they also have an organza overcoat this season which ties at the front and is very suitable, costing £170. You may also like to try cutting old cardigans to just under breast level. I did this many moons ago with an old putty-coloured scoop-neck button-front body that I had which was never any good as a body and so I cropped it really short, in essence making it into no more than a pair of sleeves. This proved to be a most useful garment while lifting baby piglets, as it was a most unobtrusive way of keeping warm (no hems trailing in pig muck). Then I started wearing it with my empire-line dress and a whole new look was born.

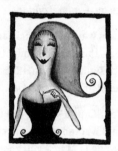

Please can you help? On the BBC2 programme *Looking Good* they showed a brief catwalk clip of a model wearing a gorgeous leather corset, which would be perfect for displaying my boobs in. Do you know where I could get a similar item that wouldn't cost the earth? Under £300 would be nice, though I know I'm probably being unrealistic. Also, any suggestions if I had such a thing as to what I could wear with it? Please don't tell me I'd look ridiculous – I'm size 10 on top, but size 12+ (depending on garment) on the bottom. – *R. Hayward, East Sussex*

Looking Good, as presented by minxy Lowri Turner, said that the one featured was by Vivienne Westwood. It's not sold off the peg but can be made to order, in leather, for loads, about £800. If you decide you want to spend that much, then go to the shop at 6 Davies Street, London w1, tel: 0171 629 3757. OK, other option: Whitaker Malem, who specialize in moulded leather, could make you a couture one, but again you'd need to go to London to have a few fittings and prices *start* at £300. Mmmm. This looks like an expensive business. Why don't you have a peekie in a magazine called *Skin 2*, which often has stuff like this at cheaper prices. As for what to wear with it, anything really – no one will be looking at anything save for your saucy leather corset.

This got some very interesting replies:

First, excuse the anonymous nature of this information, but I don't want my name linked with the Fetish Fair – my clients don't know about my secret perverted life! Anyway, your correspondent enquiring about leather corsets might like to know about the Fetish Fair who meet once a month – they are very friendly and welcoming and not at all sleazy or oppressive. There's a wide range of leather gear (whips and collars and cuffs as well as corsets!), as well as suppliers who would probably do a bespoke job for considerably less than the prices quoted in your column. Not to mention the stall selling rubber, silk, latex, canes, dildos, etc. For further info, access their website is http://www.whiplash.co.uk. – *John, London*

I've written to you before and wanted to remain anonymous. You called me Secret Man, thanks. Anyway, this company might have a leather corset for under £300 for R. Hayward: Tight Situation, PO Box 860, London SE12 OLL, tel: 0181 857 7146. – *Secret Man Again, London*

I am in love with Leonardo DiCaprio – don't you think he's just the finest thing? But aside from that, I wanted to get a necklace like Kate Winslet wore in the film, the 'Coeur de la Mer' – you know, the blue heart diamond she put on when Leo (as Jack) drew her with no clothes on. Oooh, I'm getting all hot and bothered, wish that had been me. Anyway, where can I get one? I thought it was grand. – *Jenny Pilkinton, Fleetwood*
Jenny, you want to calm down. I cannot share in your (and the rest of the world's) current obsession with Leonardo since he bears more than a passing resemblance to a controlling, insecure ex I had once and do not care to be reminded of again; but this was many moons ago, before I met my beloved. Ahhhh. So apart from the fact that DiCaprio shares a name with my eldest son and the fabulous da Vinci, no, I do not think he is the finest thing. Right then, this 'Heart of the Sea' business. This actual stone never really existed; 20th Century Fox asked Asprey's to make the costume piece of jewellery (supposedly an enormous heart-shaped blue diamond

made from the real stone stolen from the crown of Louis XVI of
Paris). Asprey's later made it up for real, but using a sapphire from
Sri Lanka as the heart, not a diamond. Anyway, I tried lashings of
places but none of the obvious people (Agatha, Butler and Wilson,
Selfridges, Harvey Nicks, Accessorize, etc.) have done one – what a
wasted marketing opportunity. So the only solution I have is for if
you are really serious about this bauble. If you are, then ring Janet
Fitch on 01932 866449 and they will select a jewellery designer to
make it; the price will vary but it will be about £400. So you really,
really need to like the little porky-looking DiCaprio.

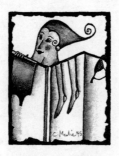

hidey-holes
how to hide the things you
don't like and show off those you do
this deals with the serious: from turbans for chemotherapy patients to the everyday problem of how to hide tummies, and also how best to show off nice things like curves

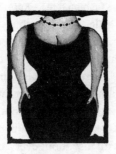

I am thirty years old, 5'7", and my statistics are 36–28–35. My legs are quite long, which means that, as well as being thick-waisted, I am short-bodied. What can I wear to disguise this awful middle of mine, as no amount of exercise seems to help? P.S. I have awful problems with evening wear. – *Juliette Wills, Devon*

Your middle is not awful in the slightest. The supposed 'ideal' is having bust and hip measurements that are the same and the waist ten inches less that this (i.e., 36, 26, 36), so yours are just a few inches off being bloody perfect, you lucky cow. You also are fairly tall with long legs. You need a good slap round the head, my dear, for there is nothing wrong with you. But anyway, you see this as a problem. What not to wear are things like baggy jumpers, which obviously have their purpose, and I'll bet you've been wearing a fair few of these in order to disguise that middle of yours. Don't. Wear lots of fitted jackets. Get any old cardigans and chop them off to just under bosom level. This defines your waist and makes your body look longer. Belts also highlight the waist (although I can't bear to wear them). Evening wear? Get your legs out, wear shimmering sheer tights and a miniskirt or hot pants (yes, really), fluff your cleavage up and forget about your waist. Your admirers will find it for you as they snake their hopeful arms around it. [God, I feel quite depressed now. I have taken to snatching chocolate *from my children's hands* as I write this book. Today I ate a creme egg before I had even entered one chapter and I am forced to hide wrappers down my *sofa's* cleavage.]

I know everyone says this to you all the time, but I really love your column. I have three problems: I have a large bosom, very small waist and the biggest bum in the world, honestly. I look best in little agnes b T-shirts, which make my chest practically disappear and show off my waist, but then I can't walk out of a room without putting on a coat to cover my bum. What should I be wearing? Are hipsters right out? Why didn't Vivienne Westwood

succeed in making bottoms fashionable? – *Kate, London*
I can't understand how little agnes b T-shirts make your chest practically disappear but it obviously works for you, so good. It is pointless me saying 'go here and buy this', since I don't think this is the sort of advice you need. There are certain things that might work for you, and here is a selection. First and most importantly, being confident about how you are is *everything*; before you sigh and say 'I know that', you obviously aren't – yet. When I was in Italy recently there was this woman with just about everything 'wrong' with her. Her upper arms were just a touch too flabby, her clothes were just a bit too tight, her bra strap was showing and she was wearing these slipper things in the street and her bottom was *enormous*. On top of all this, she had an apron on (as these Latin women tend to, you know), but by bosoms she was *sexy*. Normally I would have baulked (inwardly, silently) and thought, 'Cor, she hasn't got a clue.' But she radiated something: she was attractive, really attractive, because she was totally confident. I have to admit that for days afterwards I tried to affect this nonchalant mode of dress. Even my husband said she was one of the sexiest women he had ever met (after me, of course). But I digress. Cut-off cardigans are brilliant for you [see previous problem]. If you don't have any, buy cheap ones and cut them off yourself; they should come to just below bust level. The old trick of tying a cardigan or something else around your waist is also a good camouflage trick (make sure it is made of thin material or else you will just bulk yourself out). Vivienne Westwood did, absolutely, make bottoms fashionable. And look at Alexander McQueen's stonkingly sexy tailoring. Didn't you see Kate Winslet at the Oscars and how sexy she looked in one of his Givenchy couture outfits? (If you should ever be interested in McQueen's Givenchy couture, ring the Paris office for more details on 003 314 431 5000.) There are few things sexier than a woman with an hourglass figure.

Recently I lost all my hair due to chemotherapy but I still wish to look nice, both indoors and out. I can only bear to wear a wig for a short while and, at forty-three, turbans make me look too matronly. Square scarves are fun but I can only find polyester ones in the shops and they slide off easily. Any ideas? Please don't ask me to go bald disgracefully – it frightens my son. Thank you. – *Ruth Burrows, Bristol*
I wouldn't dream of telling you to go bald, even though I think it can look beautiful. I can't imagine how I'd feel if I lost my hair, even

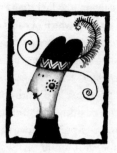

temporarily, but I can try to understand what a blow it must be to a woman's self-confidence. I don't want your son to be frightened either! I turned to the Macmillan Cancer Relief Fund, who spoke to two specialist nurses in this field on my behalf. Obviously they deal with problems such as these every day; they suggested using cotton scarves, as these don't slip as much as polyester. (My hint would also be that crêpy fabric – either silk or synthetic – would be less slippery, as the surface isn't as smooth.) They also suggested getting a stretchy Alice band and sewing your scarf to it: i.e., fold the material over the band to cover it, don't sew it all the way round, slip it on to your head and then tie the scarf at the back of your neck. Remember you can also use lengths of material, which you just need to hem. I know it's a pain sewing, but this will give you so much more choice. You might also like to experiment with light cotton hats when spring comes, but I appreciate that you may feel a little silly wearing these indoors. I know you don't like the idea of turbans or wigs, but for the sake of others in this predicament who would like to try them, Macmillan also told me about two companies. Lizannes of Luton Ltd (01323 766894) make turbans and have a great deal of expertise in this field; they cost £1.50 and members of the public can ring them direct. Then there is Natural Image Wigs, who supply department stores. They also make turbans (towelling £7 and polyester £8), in various colours; to find out details of stockists and mail order, call them on 0171 403 2440. I really hope this helps and that you make a speedy and full recovery.

I am fifty and recently retired from a job where I always wore a uniform. Suddenly I don't know what to wear. The only clothes I wore apart from my uniform were smart things (for 'dos') or really casual clothes for slobbing about. In my mind's eye I am still twenty, but of course I am not and the pear shape I had then has grown more exaggerated. I find myself thinking

of clothes I wore in my late teens (the last time I really spent any time actually thinking about my wardrobe), which of course don't suit me now! I have lots of time on my hands and am happy to spend a fair amount on clothes, but am at a loss as to what to buy. What shapes would flatter a pear shape? – *Susan, Colchester*

It will take you a while to adjust and find your natural style again, so I wouldn't recommend rushing out and buying lots of new clothes just yet. There is a temptation to wear tight bottoms and just a huge jumper all the time, and while this will hide your pear shape it doesn't give you much scope. The major mistake, I find, that pear shapes make is when buying suits, because they buy them as a whole (i.e., size 12 top and bottom), and, in order to avoid buying a huge-size jacket, the bottom half is usually a touch too tight. This will just accentuate a pear shape. If you can't buy a matching jacket and skirt/trousers in different sizes, then buy separates and stick to darker colours for your bottom half and keep the lighter colours for your top half. Also dresses that flare out from the waist or bust (empire line) will hide your bottom and show off your top. A slightly fuller skirt with a tucked-in blouse would also work well for you, but avoid too much pleating or gathering around the stomach *if* this is a problem area for you. When wearing trousers, go for a slightly flared leg. Nothing will accentuate your pear shape more than tight all-the-way-down trousers; you need a bit of width at the bottom to balance out your hips. Also, go for tops/jumpers that are short and sit on the hips, but are not too tight – if the bottoms you are wearing are tight – as again this will simply accentuate things you don't want to. Buy a couple of things and see how you go.

I have recently moved into a new flat with no cupboard space and I hate wardrobes. At the moment I have my clothes on movable rails like the ones they have in shops. It's creating a bit of an eyesore. I know this isn't a fashion problem as such, but I wondered what I could do to hide the clothes. I thought some designers like Ralph Lauren might have done nice blankets or throws that I could drape over. I don't mind spending a bit. – *Ursula Ward, Sidcup*

Yes, Ralph Lauren do some fine lifestyly things. But I think this might get on your nerves. You know, having to take the throw off every time you want to get to your McCartney dress, put it back on, take it off to look for the Berardi jacket. Then the throw/blanket thing falls off. All very annoying. I have a much better idea. Remember screens? Those great old-fashioned things that every lady used to have in her boudoir. Well, a company called Minx Design specializes in bespoke hand-crafted folding screens that are just gorgeous. Like a lot of gorgeous things, unfortunately, they do not come cheap. Prices start at £300 and go up to about £3,600 and they make the screens in the materials of your choice, so it is a piece of art as well. It takes from six to eight weeks and of course you can undress behind them, flipping your La Perla underwear over as you go, which is well sexy and mysterious. John Lewis sometimes do them in their gifts department, like Chinese painted ones for £149 or leather-look ones in red or black for £279. Bill Amberg, the leather man, can make screens using leather with wood or metal. There is one in his shop at the moment which is a whopping £2,300 + VAT and it would be made to commission and take four to six weeks; call his workshop on 0181 960 2000. I rather fancy one from Minx. Mmmmm.

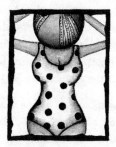

I am sixty and love swimming, which I do three times a week. I have found it impossible to replace my now clapped-out swimsuits. I am looking for the heavier weight, regular legs (not up to the waist), good bust support (not wires), preferably black or similar (i.e., not patterns). I can only find thin beach-type wear with either soft foam cups or nothing at all. I need the heavier material because of the wear and tear of local swimming pools and chemicals. I can't get much beyond central Manchester, Stockport and immediate outlying areas. Have you any ideas? Is there a mail-order firm who caters for proper *swimming* suits? I am 5'7¹/2", 38B, 29" waist, 38" hip and a size 16. I am also long-bodied. – *Josephine, Stockport, Cheshire*
Don't dismiss thin swimwear, because no matter how thick the fabric it will eventually succumb to chlorine's destructive qualities. I got through swimsuit after swimsuit and did find a thicker-than-usual one in the children's department once (which go up to remarkably big sizes, believe me; I have a big bosom and not disproportionate hips). But now I swim in a top-of-the-range Speedo ('serious'

swimwear available from department stores), which although of incredibly thin material has lasted me longer than any other. DuPont, the manufacturers of Lycra, invented the first chlorine-resistant Lycra twenty-five years ago, so make sure you look for Lycra in your swimwear as this will go some way towards helping your swim-suit last. My swimsuit has no actual support as such and I don't think it is really necessary. You might insist you do want some sort of bosom support, but the more 'serious' swimsuits do tend not to have any and by rejecting these you are eliminating a great many suitable suits. Try the Plain Jane swimsuit by Racing Green (0990 411111), which has a 'bra shelf' in the lining in two body lengths in black, navy and royal blue, is very simple and not high-cut; it costs £20 and contains Lycra. John Lewis also do a classic-design swimsuit suitable for you and there is a branch near you in Cheadle, which I hope won't be too difficult for you to get to (0161 491 4914). And Bust Stop (0181 943 9733 for a catalogue) also do a few styles of swimsuit by mail order, which might be helpful, with low legs and invisible floating wires. [Also have a look at the 'Swimwear' directory at the back of the book and especially at the entry for Splash Out, as they can make swimwear to order in the (suitable) fabric of your choice.]

This is not so much a fashion problem as one of availability and where-abouts. I am sixty-four years old, short and fat. Major surgery has necessi-tated physiotherapy, which includes swimming. Years of attempts at slimming have left me with an abdominal 'flap' and I really need support in that region. Are there any manufacturers who make swimming costumes in large sizes which give some support/control? Many years ago Spinela and Spencer did some, but I haven't heard of either of these for some time. Budget-wise, I would not wish to spend more than £50–£75 and I shop in the Harrogate, York, Leeds area. I do hope you can help. I am certain that I am not alone with this problem. – *Judith Haffenden, North Yorks*

Fantasie is a great label that does all sorts of swimwear (and under-wear) for 'problem' sizes/figures (I hate that word, but you know what I mean; they don't do just the easy-peasy swimwear that every-one else does, they tackle the problems normal people have too!). In their Classic Collection they have a selection of swimsuits with tummy control in sizes 32–44 B to G cup, approx. price £60 (for stockist enquiries, call 01536 760282). Triumph (01793 720232) have a range in their collection called Charme which provides abdominal support (due to Lycra lining on tummy). These retail from £35.

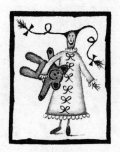

cooooosy
keeping comfortable and warm and toasty
long johns, slippers, pyjamas and fleece

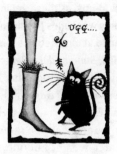

Help. I have very cold feet and my kittens, Ollie and Stanley, keep biting my toes! In the 1980s my friend Clare had some fab boot slippers which were fur-lined and may or may not have been called Ugg Boots (this is what she called them). They had a semi-hard sole (at least I think so, as I often saw her trotting about outside in them) and I think, for slippers, were quite expensive. Unfortunately, Clare has emigrated to Australia. Do they still exist? Where can I buy some? Please help!
– *Sophie Cullinan, Ramsbottom, Bury*

I am hardly surprised that your friend emigrated to Australia if that was the level of your conversation. They are now called Celt Boots and you can get in touch with the Celtic Sheepskin Co. (01637 871605), who will tell you your nearest stockist; there are lots of different styles to choose from. The Celt slippers (which, fabbily, are machine-washable) come in twenty-five colours, are sized 1–14 and cost £27.95 (+ £2 p&p).

I'm looking for men's reasonably priced pyjamas with cord-tie waist – not elastic. I've found one place in Chiswick but at £50 each can't afford to buy my dad a selection. – *name withheld, Hove, East Sussex*

Johnny Loulou branches (0171 629 7711) nearly always do some from about £25. For anyone else with a bit more to spend, Higginbotham do some with self-fabric ties (mail order: 01379 668833) – splendid pure cotton ones for £56 in four different striped colourways: red/white; blue on white; green/red on white; and white on blue. Sizes M, L and XL (they are very generously sized).

We have recently moved from a cosy London terrace to a draughty, cold heap and I am desperate to find a really WARM dressing gown. I don't want one of those horrid cheap fluffy ones that go bobbly straight away, or anything quilted like my grandma used to wear. I would like wool or wool mix if possible, ideally with a button-up neck rather than wrap-over and neat sleeves rather than huge turn-ups, as these get in the way. Harrods have quoted £300–£500 – the only wool ones I've been able to find so far – too much for me. I could pay up to about £120 or so. Maybe a dressmaker could make me one? – *Sarah Hollis, Sunningdale, Berks*

Well, you certainly could look through the 'Dressmaker' directory if you want to, but otherwise get yourself along to Selfridges, who do a lovely one, Vald'arizes, in Pyrenean style, with a hood and zip (not button-up, I know, but nice all the same), in wool and cashmere, £155. Or try a winter-weight kimono, in silk or cotton (silk is very warm, remember). Asahi, at 110 Golbourne Road, London W10 5PS, do some beautiful vintage ones from the 1920s–1960s: their bargain bin has ones up to £20, others are up to £70, and you will have something totally original. Call them on 0181 960 7299, as they can also do mail order.

I have recently worn out a favourite nightshirt and am finding it impossible to replace. My requirements are that it must be brushed cotton and it must be full (calf/ankle) length, preferably with only three or four buttons at the neck, like a rugby shirt, not buttons all the way down. I would rather that it did not have a collar. All of the nightshirts that I have been able to find in London have been like big shirts: buttons all the way down, with a big floppy collar and not nearly long enough (barely to the knee). Is there anywhere I could get one more like the one that has gone into holes? (The old one had 'Bonsoir, Made in England' on the label and came from an outfitters in Oxford, if that helps.) – *J. W. Stevenson, London WC1*

You fusspot! But luckily, help is at hand. Bonsoir make fabulous pyjamas and night stuff; my father always wears them and when I was very small I used to wear his pyjama tops when he went away on business because they smelt of him. Hence I have always had a bit of a soft spot for Bonsoir (call 0171 439 2101 and they will send a catalogue straight away). They do brushed-cotton nightshirts in the winter and plain cotton in the summer. They cost about £55 and are calf-length. Hopefully this will provide you with exactly what you want.

My husband had always loved galoshes, or gentlemen's overshoes as I think they are known these days. He bought his last pair at a small shop in Grasmere about twelve years ago, but when he went back the premises had been turned into an ice-cream parlour. We live on a damp hillside in one of the wettest areas in Britain and galoshes are a lot more comfortable

than wellingtons for pastoral visiting, which, being a vicar, my husband does a lot. Please, please, can you help track down someone who sells these useful items? If so, you would turn his mourning into joy!
– *Val Haynes, Halifax*

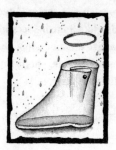

Galoshes can be obtained from Wagstaff (01484 683233) for under £10. Others to try are Ernest Draper & Co. (01604 752609), Worrell Bros (0181 959 1647) and R. C. Smith's in Greenock (01475 888555). So Reverend Haynes should be happy now. Remember us all in your prayers, Revd!

Once upon a time there was a Japanese shop in Brighton and there I once bought a cotton kimono which I have used as a summer dressing gown ever since. It is cool, elegant, easily laundered and WORN OUT. So can you suggest where I might find a replacement before next year's heat wave? – *Brenda Heasman, West Sussex*

You must visit Asahi in London (10 Golbourne Road, London w10 5ps, tel: 0181 960 7299) if you can [see Sarah's letter above]. They specialize in vintage kimonos, with some dating back to the early nineteenth century. They have hundreds of different designs, colours and fabrics: rayon, silk, cotton; and they're all handmade. It is the perfect place for anyone wanting to pick up something slightly different in the dressing-gown department. Cotton ones are more modern but are still not new. Prices start at £10. Bargain! Although, like all lovely things, you have to see them. If you really don't want to make the trip, you can call Asahi up and be really specific about the sort of thing you want and they may be able to satisfy you postally.

I think that the kimono that your correspondent is looking for is actually what the Japanese call a *yukata* – a sort of dressing gown that people are given when they stay at traditional hotels. A kimono is a much more formal

garment and not normally washable. I used to live in Brighton and recall the Japanese shop sold both. I have a couple of *yukata*s which were both bought in Japan. If your correspondent wants one, I would suggest that the shops in the Yaohan Plaza, on the Edgware Road in London, are worth a look – it's a large Japanese shopping centre. Alternatively, try Japanese department stores in London like Sogo in Piccadilly (0171 333 9000). Do watch the sizing – the Japanese are much smaller than the British. I (at 5'7") bought a men's garment in Japan. I hope this helps. I think your column (and the 'Big Shoe' directory) is great!
– *Susie Northfield, Didcot*

Thanks for the very helpful advice, Susie, and the compliments. More please.

I need some sort of trainers with a Velcro fastening. They're good for me because I'm always in a hurry when I go swimming in the morning, and they're good for my eighty-five-year-old mum, who has mobility problems. Tying laces can be quite a problem. Clarks used to make them (in adult sizes) but my local shoe shop tells me it's only possible to get them in children's sizes now. Many thanks. – *Norma Herdson, Maidenhead*

OK, Norma, try this lot: Smart Shoe Saver, Harrington Dock, Liverpool L70 1AX. They cost £5.95 per pair and are available in ladies' sizes 3–8. Between 8.30 a.m. and 10 p.m. they can be contacted on 0151 709 8909. There is a charge for p&p and insurance of £3.95. The Clifford James catalogue has a few Velcro-fastening shoes (call 0990 230303), and try Sander & Kay, Mail Order House, China Lane, Manchester M99 1SA (enquiries: 0161 236 5555). K shoes have Mercury Velcro-fastening trainers, £21.99 for adult sizes (enquiries: 0990 785886). And finally, try the Bright Life UK catalogue (0151 709 8909).

I would be most grateful if you could save me a trip to Tokyo and the expense incurred. You see, I'm after a full-length Puffa-type jacket – one that goes all the way down to my ankles – and the only people I've seen wearing them are Japanese. There was one exception, but he was a musician who had been on tour in Japan. The coat I'm looking for also has a big sculpted hood, but it is otherwise plain. It is the coolest-looking coat I have ever seen and doubtless one of the warmest too. But where, oh where, can I find one? It's not fair – all these Japanese students (probably at St Martin's) are always immaculately dressed and seem to get the coolest clothes. – *Guy, via e-mail (Oxford)*

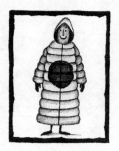

I picked yours to answer but I have had twelve enquiries about this
sort of coat. You can get them here. They are made by Windcoat
and sold in Selfridges, Harrods, Fenwicks, Liberty, Pollyanna in
Barnsley (those are the stockists; none nearer you but, for goodness' sake, you're not far from London). Prices start at £215 (not
that expensive really, considering we are talking a designer label
here) and they come in loads of colours. Although it is a 'women's
range' don't be put off – most styles are dead simple, unisex, some
styles zip up and lots of men buy them (enquiries: 0171 730 1234).
Some do have a hood but it tends to be zipped away. Soviet do a
men's one, three-quarter-length, in lots of colours, £180 (enquiries
0171 839 4455). I have a feeling these are going to become very
popular, however, so by the time you read this I'll bet every Tom
has done one.

**I'm looking for a winter dressing gown that's warm yet has a touch of
glamour. All the department stores offer a choice between wispy silk,
which is quite unsuitable for an English winter, or warm but dull and
grannyish gowns. Any suggestions? – Liz, London**
You have not mentioned a price limit, but Margaret Howell has
done the most divine velvet robes in charcoal or black for £295 for
silk velvet (very warm) or £195 for cotton velvet. Margaret Howell
has shops at 29 Beauchamp Place, London SW3 1NJ, and 24 Brook
Street, London W1Y 1AE (enquiries: 0171 584 2462). Connolly (0171
235 3883) do some fabulous ones, cashmere for £1,300, cotton,
linen for £400. Or you could do as my friend Lily Vermouth does:
of a morning she always sticks a tiara on her head; that way even if
she answers the door in an old candlewick button-up jobbie, she
looks fantastic.

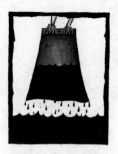

dry-cleaning dramas
and wet-cleaning ones too,
as well as dyeing things you're sick of
*anything and everything to do
with washing and dyeing*

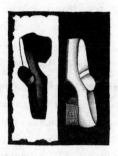

I have a pair of white leather loafers which I wore quite a lot in the summer, but am loath to get rid of them, even though I know they will be quite passé by next summer. They are still in good repair, so is it sensible to dye them black, to get some winter wear out of them, and if so how would you recommend going about it? They have a 1" heel in pale, varnished wood.
– *Susie Thomson, East Sheen*

You are right to dye them. Dyeing, whether it be shoes or clothes, is an easy and cheap way to revitalize your wardrobe and a trick that not enough people make use of. Dylon Shoe Colour make a whole heap of dyes for shoes, in lots of colours to suit leather, synthetic and canvas shoes. It costs £2.45 and gives a long-lasting finish that doesn't crack or peel (they also do a Satin Shoe Colour for £1.95). Dylon have also given me a handy hint to create a mock-croc effect you may like to try, which involves painting the dye over an orange netting bag. As for the heel, this shouldn't look odd. But if you decide you don't like it you could either paint the heels (get one of those little pots from your DIY or art shop, making sure it is suitable for wood), you can stain them with wood stain, or you could try just brushing black shoe polish into them. I find this is sometimes enough to darken the heel. Dylon have a brilliant consumer advice line that can help with any aspect of dyeing shoes or clothes with their dyes (0181 663 4296).

I had a dress made for me and I don't know what to do now that it needs cleaning as obviously it has no care label. – *E. Harper (Miss), Fulham*

Do you remember where you bought the fabric from? If you do, take the dress back to the shop and they may be able to tell you or give you the manufacturer's address to write to for care advice. If you or your dressmaker has scraps of fabric left, you can also take them to any reputable dry-cleaners, who will be able to test the scraps with the different dry-cleaning chemicals they use. If none of the above applies, try a top-class dry-cleaners such as Lilliman and Cox (0171 629 4555) or Tothills (0171 252 0100), as they are both very helpful and will be able to advise you.

I have a very favourite suit which feels like corded silk but the fabric is 52 per cent cupro and 48 per cent viscose. It is so comfortable and fits well, but I am not happy with the colour, which is a rather sugary pink. Would it be suitable for dyeing? If so, are there any specialists whom I should contact to carry out the job? If the fabric is unsuitable for dyeing, what would your suggestions be to achieve a different look. It has a knee-length pencil skirt and long-line waisted jacket with short sleeves.
– Elizabeth Willsher, Maldon, Essex

I keep meaning to get loads of things dyed, but haven't managed to be that organized so far. Now then, Chalfont Dyers and Cleaners, 222 Baker Street, London NW1 5RT, tel: 0171 935 7316, are apparently the people to go to. They will dye clothes and soft furnishings made from natural fibres only (cotton, silk, wool). Customers must send garments to the above address; when the garments have been assessed (age, history, etc.), paperwork will be sent out, as the customer's signature is required to go ahead with the job (which takes three to six weeks). There are about six colours available for clothes and prices vary: jumpers cost around £40, jeans £35. Their advice about your suit is that they would never dye structured jackets because the front seams can be too tiny and split in the delicate process involved. Also linings and interfacing cause too many problems. Your skirt (52 per cent cupro and 48 per cent viscose) can be dyed as both fabrics come from natural fibres, but both become limp after the dyeing process, which loses the 'dressing' somewhat. So, in short, best leave it this time. As for a different look, well . . . what, really? Wear the jacket with something else? [Look in my 'Dressmakers' directory and then you can get the suit copied and the dressmaker might be able to find the same type of fabric for you, but in a different colour.]

Why is it that after a few (machine) washes all my white underwear goes grey? And should I wash my bras by hand? – Hermione Phillips, Winchester
My guess is that you are washing them at too high a temperature. This is easy to do with whites as you bung them in the machine at about sixty degrees. They should really be washed at no higher than fifty degrees (that ten degrees less makes all the difference),

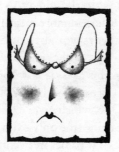

especially if they contain synthetic fibres, as most do nowadays. If a great deal of your underwear is white, then it is worth doing them in a separate delicates load (if your machine has a half-wash button then use that too if the load is small). Yes, you *should* wash your bras by hand, but who can really be bothered? They are so small and fiddly that you end up scrubbing your hands to kingdom come. And anyway people say you should change your bras every year, so what's the point? My advice is that life is too short to hand-wash anything but the most delicate of apparel. Get a laundry bag (white big netty thing, Johnny Loulou sell them), stick your bras in there, put the machine on and go and drink more gin.

I have a lovely pair of shoes that I bought for my wedding and have not worn since. They are made of a white material that looks like (but isn't) raw silk. I would like to have them dyed a cream colour (if possible) or another colour to go with an outfit (yet to be decided) for a friend's wedding in the summer. How does one set about getting this done?
– Sian Forbes, Westbury, Wiltshire
Now then, pay attention, everybody: Julia Taylor dyes shoes any colour (she mixes her own), but you need to post your shoes and a piece of fabric in the desired colour to her. Julia thinks your shoes sound like dupion silk, but would need more specific information to assess whether they can be dyed or not. Anyway, prices start at £30 (all enquiries to 0171 289 3966).

Last year, while pregnant, I splashed out on a lovely empire-line Ghost dress (£160), which was perfect then. Now, it is far too big for me (it makes me look like a hippie), yet I'd like to get more wear out of it. Also it is white and therefore slightly see-through. I thought dyeing it might also be an option. Will it make the dress shrink? – *I. Pronto (Mrs), Sheffield*
All Ghost clothes are brilliant for pregnant women because they are easy to wear and their style (flowing and empire line, wide

trousers and the like) is perfectly suited to a big tummy. They are also infinitely more stylish than most specialist maternity labels, which is why they are always worn by models pre, during and after pregnancy. Although Ghost clothes are meant to be loose, I can understand that perhaps this dress is now too big for you. As Ghost garments are all viscose-based, they are perfect for dyeing. Try Dylon's Machine Dye, which gives excellent results and it's all done in the washing machine (the only extra ingredient you'll need is salt), so there's no mess. It comes in twenty-two different colours and costs £4.35 from department stores; Dylon have a very helpful consumer advice line if you have any queries (0181 663 4296). The dress will not shrink further as it has already been shrunk in the manufacturing process, although a Ghost representative tells me that excessive tumble-drying might make it shrink slightly! Dye it first and see what happens: a darker colour might help to make it look less voluminous. Otherwise have it altered by a local dress-maker [see 'Dressmakers' directory].

I recently bought a pure-cotton sweater of a good make. Unfortunately, it is a size too big, and as I bought it in a sale and it was the last one I can't return it. Is there any method of shrinking? I don't mind taking a bit of a chance! – *James, North Yorks*

The only thing you can do is try putting it through a boil wash. But I doubt it will make any difference. Wear it a size too big – it'll look cute and girls will want to mother you. Or send it to Pavarotti, he can use it as a skinny rib.

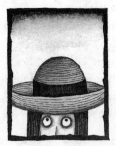

About six or seven years ago, a dear friend made me buy a straw hat which quickly became indispensable. It is made of very fine and flexible woven straw. It goes with everything I own and never blows off. Unfortunately, it is really looking its age and in need of cleaning. Is there a remedy for this? Please help. – *Catherine Rose, Olney, Bucks*

Apologies for taking so long to reply to this. I spoke to a friendly milliner, Lucy Barlow (14 Portobello Green Arcade, 281 Portobello Road, London W10 5TX, tel: 0181 968 5333), who suggested the following: pad the hat so that it isn't flat and is supported – you can use clean cotton 'rags' or tissue for this. Then get another cotton rag and rub some soap on it (you must make sure that the soap doesn't have bleach in it, otherwise the straw will go yellow – always do a patch test first, as the saying goes) and then gently go over the hat to clean it. Then, with the hat still padded out, put a clean piece of cotton over it and iron the hat. To do this it is really important that the hat is supported and not flat, so with the stuffing in the hat, put one hand in the hat and use the other to press the iron (with the cotton in between hat and iron). As long as you have this fabric to protect your hat, the iron can be quite hot. This will steam your hat back into shape. It is also really important that you don't get the hat too wet, otherwise you will ruin it. Then I also spoke to John Boyd's (0171 589 7601), a very traditional milliner's with over fifty years' experience. They clean hats, so if you're ever in London you could pop in and see them. It's difficult for either of them to say what is possible, or how much it would cost, until they see the hat, but prices for cleaning start at £15. You may decide the cost isn't worth it and instead want to buy a new one. But you obviously really like this hat, so it may be worth spending more on revamping it than it cost in the first place!

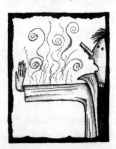

I recently bought a silver-coloured Schott pilot's jacket which cost me nearly £150 – but I thought it was well worth it as it was very warm and comfortable and even, I was told, fireproof. About four weeks later I took it to be dry-cleaned for the first time. When I collected it from the shop it smelt terribly of fried onions and I said it would need to be recleaned. When it came back again it smelt fine. The trouble is that over the last few

weeks the fried-onion smell has gradually come back. I can only assume
that it has something to do with the dry-cleaning process. What am I to do?
If I go out wearing it my friends and colleagues will think that I hang
around cheap hamburger stalls. Can you help? – *Iain, London*

I spoke to Schott's head office in New Jersey, USA, who said they
don't do a fireproof jacket. Harrods (who stock Schott) said that
the fabric content of your jacket is 50 per cent nylon and 50 per
cent rayon on the outside, with 100 per cent nylon lining. The
padding is 100 per cent polyester fibre-fill. Dr Richard Neil at the
Dry Cleaning Technology Centre was very helpful. He said that
unusual smells are a common problem when it comes to dry-
cleaning complaints. Yours sounds like (and obviously he can only
speculate) it is due to a cleaning error, where there had been a
chemical breakdown in the solvent used (this would account for
the immediate ponginess). Or, as the smell also came back gradually, it could be due to the fabric finish (i.e., manufacturing fault).
Either way, try asking your dry-cleaner to use a different machine
from the one they used previously. If the problem persists, take
the jacket back to where you bought it, explain what has happened
and they should send it back to Schott.

My student daughter recently bought a lined white linen shift dress.
Inevitably someone spilt a drink on it when she wore it to a club. As the care
label said 'Dry Clean Only', I took it to TWO dry-cleaners, both of whom said
they couldn't do anything about the stain because their stain removers
couldn't be used on linen, and they wouldn't recommend washing. Is there
anything we can do to salvage this? And isn't it time manufacturers started
making clothes that could be worn and washed without major trauma? Or at
least provided clear and prominent warnings on their more vulnerable garments? Over the last few months I've had to return at least three garments
which have shrunk or whose colours have run, and the assistants look at me
as if I'm beneath contempt for even bothering to return items which they
seem to think should be worn once and thrown away.
– *Jeannette King, Aberdeen*

I agree it is frustrating, but I am not sure what you mean about
providing 'clear and prominent warnings on their more vulnerable
garments'. Any fabric in white is 'vulnerable' and accidents do, of
course, happen. I am astonished that two dry-cleaners said they
couldn't help – linen is hardly difficult. I could understand it if you
were presenting them with a hand-beaded evening gown! And I

have never heard of stain removers not being able to be used on linen; it is a natural fibre and hardly volatile. I spoke to the woman who owns the store your daughter's dress is from and she in turn spoke to the Dry Cleaning Technology Centre, which is strictly for the trade and does not deal with enquiries from scussy members of the public. They suggest finding a dry-cleaners that uses Aquatex as a stain remover, which they say is available in better dry-cleaners. I rang the DTC for you to find out a bit more about it and see if they knew of a dry-cleaners that uses Aquatex in your area. They were uninterested in trying to help, saying they were 'rather busy' and put the phone down without so much as a 'I'm a rude pig and no mistake'. Good manners are so important. What hope is there? I have had a few letters about the great dry-cleaning debate and there are certain things that we have to understand. One is that anything with an acetate lining, no matter what the outer fabric is made from, will have to be dry-cleaned. As we strive for newer fabrics and more fancy clothes, we have to accept that they need a different level of care. But if you have cleaned any clothes according to the label instructions and they have shrunk or whatever, complain and don't stop at the assistants. Write to the head office or manager (not to me!) and demand justice.

An apology: In the above letter I mentioned the Dry Cleaning Technology Centre and said that the person who picked up the phone had been most unhelpful and put the phone down without so much as an 'I'm a rude pig and no mistake'. I'd like to apologize unreservedly to pigs everywhere, but especially those on my farm, who since this column appeared have been refusing to roll around in mud and have been snorting at me in a most unappealing fashion. In the light of mad cow disease and reported mad lamb disease, my pigs are a valuable commodity. So Hermès pig collars all round to my herd and soz soz soz.

Please help! My Prada tote bag is beginning to look old and battered. I can't afford a new one (my boyfriend won't give me his credit card), so is there a service where I can get it cleaned and shaped to its original beautiful form? – Anna, Stoke-on-Trent

Anna, Anna, Anna, all *sorts* of comments come to mind here: starving children; cures for cancer; hospital waiting lists; old people and broken hips; not enough books in schools; not enough meadows in the countryside; over-population; shrinking icecaps; Prada bags, bit

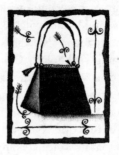

passé. Et cetera. Not to mention expecting your boyfriend to cough up. But where would the world be without nylon frippery? Anyhoo, I stuck an aubergine in my mouth and rang the Prada shop. I was rather flabbergasted to hear that they DO NOT provide a cleaning or a reshaping service – 'Nothing lasts for ever,' they said. (Miuccia, Miuccia: *che vergonia!* I must have a word with you about this next time we are having pasta e funghi sotto olio together.) They do, however, recommend Scovies (35 Dulwich Village, London SE21 7BN, tel: 0181 693 2755), where they send all Prada clothes and accessories for cleaning (I'm not sure what they mean by this as they don't provide a cleaning service . . .). Scovies clean each bag individually – no dry-cleaning – and this costs between £15 and £50 depending on bag, trimmings, etc. No chance of reshaping (apparently bags should be kept like shoes – stuffed when not in use). I also rang the TSA (Textile Services Association) on 0181 863 7755 to find cleaners registered in Stoke, and they had four. If your bag is nylon, try the Sketchley Dry Cleaners, 38 Gaolgate Street, Stafford, tel: 01785 258908. They will do it if there's a care label which says dry-cleaning is poss. It will cost about £5. If there's any plastic on it they won't because it will be ruined – they recommended bringing it in for them to have a look at. For cleaning purposes you could also try saddle soap. But otherwise it looks like you'll have to flash your boyfie and steal his wallet while he's still in shock.

In Venice in January I bought a pair of super black sheeny-shiny leather shoes. They are, however, definitely NOT patent leather, but I do want to maintain their glossy look and have as yet dared not polish them. Will ordinary polish dull the leather? Please advise. I remain, your faithful reader. – *Margot Beard, Rhodes University, Grahamstown, South Africa*
Meltonian (01753 523971) do some products (All Leather Shine

Aerosol, £3.00, or there's a 'super shine sponge', £1.49) but these products are only available in the UK. In South Africa try Kiwi products like Kiwi Elite Liquid (call them in Natal: 719 7111). Mr White at posh cobblers John Lobb said that good polish shouldn't dull the leather and that although it was difficult to say without seeing the leather, if you spend long enough – sometimes a few hours (!) – then any leather should polish up, and some traditional cobblers will polish your shoes for a fee. He gave this advice on polishing technique: all leather needs feeding, so you should push in a small amount of leather cream in small circles, adding a little bit of water as you're going round as this hardens the polish more quickly and helps to get a shine faster (like old-fashioned spit and polish). After you've worked the cream in, leave for ten minutes and then polish. If you want extra gloss, then add a wax polish to enhance the shine. Yum.

I was really pleased with myself when I found a Christian Dior suit in a second-hand shop at a third of its price new. However, I now find that it picks up stains so easily that I'm spending a fortune on dry-cleaning. It is bright red and made of pure new wool. Even a splash of water leaves a brownish stain that looks like coffee has been spilt on it. Can you suggest anything? Please keep me anonymous as I don't think anyone in my office knows I buy second-hand clothes! – D., Wiltshire

Oh, really! What shame is there in buying second-hand clothes? Rather canny and clever, I think! There is nothing I can suggest, *tant pis* (that's French), but what a pain, eh? Probably why someone bunged it in the second-hand shop in the first place. Teflon is now used as a fibre coating to aid in resisting stains but there's not very much you can do with it now . . . sorry. Donate it back to the charity shop and let someone else have the problem. Tee hee.

What is it with dry-clean-only labels? Why the epidemic? Is it laziness or fear of litigation that makes so many manufacturers slap them on even per- fectly washable fabrics? Or are they shareholders in the dry-cleaning industry? Is it a sales ploy to make us feel pampered? In any case, they're making a big mistake. I refuse to buy everyday separates which claim to require professional dry-cleaning – unless common sense tells me I can wash them, which it often has. However, I have just bought a beige, dry- clean-only microfibre mac which I'd dearly love to wash but daren't. It's 100 per cent polyester and the lining is 100 per cent acetate. My friend has a

microfibre coat she throws into the washing machine. Surely you can't get more washable than pure polyester – or can you? Is there an independent advisory body or person I could ask? Or do you know the answer? And will someone please persuade manufacturers to tell the truth about their fabrics so we can make our own minds up about how to damn well clean them? – *C. Mohr (Ms), London*

There isn't an independent advisory body or person you can ask; it's down to common sense and trial and error, I'm afraid. I have long suspected that manufacturers stick 'dry-clean' instructions in willy-nilly but trying to get anyone to admit to it is impossible. I turned to Mr Tebbs, who is MD of the Fabric Care Research Association, for a bit of advice. He said that whether a garment can be dry-cleaned or washed will very much depend on its total make-up, which must include not only the outer fabric and the lining, but any interlining, any adornments such as buttons or trims, and the appropriate dyestuffs that have been used. (This is why one thing made out of polyester might be washable and another won't be.) They advised looking for proper care labels (i.e., not just 'dry-clean only'). Believe it or not, the use of care labelling in the UK remains voluntary, so we are actually lucky to get anything at all. Some things of course do have to be dry-cleaned, either because of the fabric or because of the structure (tailored items, things with linings or shoulder pads, etc.). But while few people mind getting special-occasion clothes dry-cleaned, it is particularly annoying when you buy something that you plan to wear extensively – a slip dress or unlined pair of trousers, for example – only to find it is dry-clean only. I dry-clean nothing other than coats or posh stuff and refuse, like you, to buy anything that is dry-clean only. Of course you *can* wash lots of dry-clean-only garments perfectly successfully – I have – but the risk is ours. (Be careful with garments listing rayon or viscose in them; they can seem perfectly washable but often shrink, so follow the label instructions carefully here.) I wouldn't wash your mac, because it's not as simple as saying that this or that fibre is washable (and polyester is a fibre not a fabric), because it depends on lots of scientific stuff. And as anything with a lining does not tend to take to water, you may find the outer fabric washes well and the lining shrinks, for example. If everyone avoided dry-clean-only clothes wherever possible and *wrote* to the shops and manufacturers to make their point, things might change rather quicker.

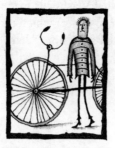

My problem is this: how can I bring back the 'puff' back into my 'puffa'? Being a keen all-weather city cyclist, my favoured outer garment is the puffa jacket, which is deliciously warm and practical in the winter. Sadly, however, it seems that after no more than two seasons' use the macho Michelin look evaporates and I am left with a limp rag that hangs and droops dull and lifeless. All of these treasures are goose down-filled and three have a nylon exterior. The most expensive one is a £500 leather Schott puffa, which I am naturally loath to replace. Washing one once in a machine, I have discovered this to be completely ruinous and I doubt that dry-cleaning will rejuvenate them. Is there a cure? How can I reintroduce the zest and spring into my poorly puffas?

– Ken Russell, London

Are you *the* Ken Russell? Now then, there is a make called Puffa, but this is often used as a generic to describe all those jackets. I called Puffa and they said that if it were a real Puffa then it would be filled with exclusive Puffa down – which is fully machine-washable. Goose down hasn't been used in their jackets for over ten years – they could only suggest taking it to a dry-cleaners for special cleaning advice. I then spoke to the manageress at Hayward Dry Cleaners, 25b Lowndes Street, London SW1X 9JF, tel: 0171 235 4844, who was a delight and said that if you take it in the fabric consultant would look into the possibilities of restuffing (might be worth it for the leather one), but it would depend on technicalities like the stitching, etc. I then rang Schott for a second opinion and they said an interesting thing: put your non-leather jackets in a cool wash (I know you've tried this before but . . .) of forty degrees with a clean trainer in there as well to agitate the wash and fluff up the feathers! But don't tumble-dry. For the leather one just shake it around a lot . . . mmm, not sure about how useful this piece of advice is! You may be interested to know that there are things called Washballs made by Pure Tech (01482 322506 for catalogue or to order) which do this fluffing-up business and have been tested so as not to harm delicate fabrics; you get two for £16.50.

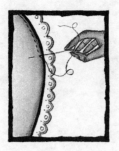

sew, sew
making and mending
old stuff becomes new again

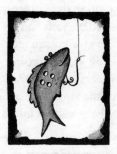

Two years ago at a Nicole Farhi sale I bought a skirt and jacket suit with divine pewter fish-shaped buttons. I have now lost one of them and am distraught. Can I find fish-shaped buttons anywhere else? Should I change the whole lot? – *Karen Hamilton, London*

I spoke to Nicole Farhi's office for you and they said that they keep a 'button box' with buttons from past collections, so although they can't promise to have your button you're in with a good chance. Ring the manageress of the Bond Street shop and she'll put you in touch with the appropriate person (0171 499 8368). It is this sort of sterling after-sales service which makes buying British designer clothes worthwhile. Just in case they don't have your button and you decide to change all of them, you may wish to try the Button Queen, 19 Marylebone Lane, London WIM 5FE (0171 935 1505); this shop has a smorgasbord of buttons for you to choose from.

My husband's ageing Barbour jacket has got its zip stuck and we can't shift it. This is particularly annoying as I wear it most and it was only when he put it on for some gardening in the rain that the zip decided to misbehave. It seems to be one notch out of sync and won't unfasten at either end. Do Barbour run a repairs service for eleven-year-old jackets, or could anyone else do something about it? Handy phone numbers, addresses, etc. would be gratefully received. – *Kate Marsh, Dorset*

Yes, Barbour do run a repairs service – in fact, they have a very sophisticated after-sales service (good-quality, performance labels such as Barbour and Burberry do, you'll find, offer good after-sales service, which makes the initial outlay worth it). They reproof, repair and make alterations to nearly 1,000 of their waxed-cotton jackets every week. The Customer Service Department tell me that they have received jackets dating back to the 1930s, so your eleven-year-old jacket will be no problem to them. You should send your husband's jacket, with a note explaining the problem and your address and telephone number, to Customer Service Department, J. Barbour and Sons, Simonside, South Shields, Tyne and Wear NE34 9PD, tel: 0191 455 4444. To give you an idea, your jacket would cost £33.25 inclusive of VAT and p&p to replace the zip and reproof it (a good idea after eleven years); separately this is £18.75 for the reproofing and £14.50 for the zip. These are standard prices; more fanciness will cost more. They will require payment before carrying out the work.

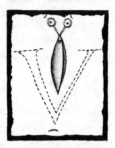

This request is slightly at a tangent to your usual queries, but I hope you'll be able to help. I make most of my clothes and love dressmaking. Thanks to Vogue patterns, I could have a wardrobe full of Donna Karan and Issey Miyake, but finding fabric is depressingly difficult. Liberty is fantastic, but I wonder if you could suggest anywhere a bit closer to Leeds, or mail-order specialists. I've tried finding shops through magazine adverts, but without much success. What I'm after at the moment are wool/Lycra mixes, wool jersey, cotton duck and trouser-weight linen. Any suggestions would be greatly appreciated. – *Sue Hamelman, Leeds*

The good news is that Liberty produce a catalogue which costs £3.50 + 50p p&p, but this does not have everything in it. For other stuff they can also provide samples of fabrics if you contact them: Liberty, Regent Street, London W1R 6AH, tel: 0171 734 1234 (ask for extension 2244 for the mail-order catalogue). John Lewis, Oxford Street, London W1A 1EX, tel: 0171 629 7711 (ask for dress fabrics), also provide a spiffing service, which is nothing less than I would expect of my beloved Johnny Loulou (and no this isn't an advert). They have a whole department dedicated to samples! And will send out, free of charge, up to five samples of fabric if you call and describe the sort of thing you want. This is for fabric up to £25 per metre; any fabric costing more than that and you will have to buy a ten-centimetre piece. When you have decided what you want, you can order by phone, paying by Switch or account card (not credit cards). Allans, 75 Duke Street, London wıм 5dj, tel: 0171 629 5947, don't have a catalogue but if you write in explaining what you want, with an SAE, they will then select several suitables and send them out. They keep a note of the reference number of what they've sent, so if you decide 'Yes please!' they know what you're referring to and then you can order and pay by cheque/credit card. Nevtext Interloop Ltd on 0115 959 8781 are mail-order merchants with a very simple catalogue that is nevertheless stuffed full of fabrics and trimmings, mostly for dance and theatrical use (they tend to be bright). Prices vary wildly but you can buy whatever amount you want, although it works out cheaper if you buy in bulk.

I have a lovely pale yellow cotton jumper with some cabling and decorative ribbing at the cuffs and bottom. But I have been unable to wear it for a while as, despite careful washing, it has stretched to ridiculous proportions. Although still OK in width, its length now reaches my knees and the sleeves flap around about 5" beyond my fingertips. Is there any way I can successfully shorten it again? I am very handy at sewing but to date have been afraid of taking the scissors to it for fear of ruining it altogether. Please don't suggest I wear it as a dress as that would look very silly on me. Perhaps you and your panel of experts can come up with a solution for me?
– *Cathy Sweeny, Dublin*

Why don't you wear it as a dress? Joke! This business of 'you and your panel of experts' – there isn't one, there is just me. I have assistants sometimes, for a few days here and there, but then I miss the research, the detective work, as I track things down and the thrill of it all, and I drive them mad with my nit-picking, 'Have you tried there, or there, or here?' or 'Look in there and through that', and I can see them thinking, 'Do it yourself, then.' So I do. Before you heed my advice, you must realize that I cannot take responsibility for anything going wrong, OK? The proper way to do it is to unravel the yarn until it is the length that you want it to be, then you need to go round with a crochet hook and secure the stitches. It is impossible for me to describe this to you (and I don't actually know how to do it, as my mamma always does it for me), so I suggest you find a friend who is good with a crochet hook and get her/him to show you. The other, very irresponsible thing I've done is cut a jumper, then with a big needle threaded with some spare yarn that you take from the severed bit, sew the hem up, catching the stitches as you go. But remember that you will end up with a plain hem that most probably flares out because you have removed the rib. As it's a shop-bought knit, I doubt you will be able to reproduce the rib yourself by hand-knitting it. Find an old aunt somewhere, shove it in her direction and give her a digestive biscuit and a cup of tea. I've been no help at all, have I?

I have a beloved envelope briefcase that my parents gave me and it is in very good nick, but the zip is starting to go – the fabric part is tearing, it is quite old. I love this briefcase but now use it only for special occasions. Where can I get the zip fixed? – A., London

Although I've never taken anything there myself, a reader recommended Michael's Shoe Care at 10/12 Procter Street, London WC1V 6NX, tel: 0171 405 7436. They also have branches at Ludgate Hill, Liverpool Street and Fenchurch Street. They repair zips on bags for a flat fee of £19.95.

I am writing to you as I have all sorts of problems when I am buying suits. The jackets nearly always fit, but the trousers are always much more of a problem – I think that I must have a very strange shape. As a result I have in the past used a tailor in Watford – S. Leonard (very excellent man) – and this has been fine. However, I have recently moved to Northampton, and I shall have to find another tailor now. My problem is finding the material. I would like to be able to go directly to the manufacturers and then take the material to the tailor to be made up into suits. I would appreciate any help that you can give me in this area, as I have been unable to locate any manufacturers of suit cloth – though I am sure that there must be many in the country. – Simon May, via e-mail

Well, any good tailor should be able to offer you a selection of fabric. I don't know of any tailors in Northampton, I'm afraid. As for fabrics: Jasons of Bond Street represent men's tailoring companies – so they have over 1,000 swatches to choose from and once you've chosen, the fabric will be there in no time (between one hour and two days). You can even choose by phone. Ring 0171 629 2606 and describe the type of fabric you want: i.e., winter-weight pinstripe. They will select ten-ish suitable fabrics (although this isn't relevant to you I thought I'd mention that they won't send out lace samples because of the amount needed to see the pattern) and send the swatches to you; you then send back the one you want. You can buy any amount, from the length of a suit leg upwards, and as they are good-quality fabrics they will typically cost £60 per metre for an autumn/winter-weight fabric. Pay by credit card over the phone and it will be delivered to you, or you can pick it up. Liberty does the same thing; there is a charge for payment depending on weight. Prices are roughly £40 per metre for suiting fabric but can go up to £800 per metre; for a suit you'd probably need three metres, so £2,400 for top-quality cashmere. Call 0171 734 1234, extension 2244, for mail-order department. If it's too specialized for them, they'll refer you to the appropriate department. Allans, 75 Duke Street, London WIM 5DJ, tel: 0171 629 5947 [see Sue's problem earlier on in this chapter] should be able to help.

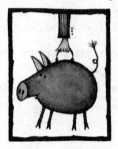

I am desperate to find a supply source for a replacement hand-grip on my suede pigskin attaché case – German manufacture but unspecified, therefore metric size. I understand that there is a high-quality luggage repairer in London, any details please. – *John, Swansea*

Ay, John, you don't like to go in for too much chittie-chat, do you? Very to the point and curt. Hope you're not like that when chatting up prospective romantic partners. Selfridges in London's Oxford Street (0171 629 1234) have a luggage repair concession in store that has been there for going on two and ten year and it is very popular. They said that in principle they could do it but in practice they'd have to see it. They have a lot of handles in stock but they'd have to find the right size and the right colour for the case. There is a £10 minimum charge for fitting and *sometimes* this £10 also includes the handle; it depends on what you want. Generally, prices depend on lots of things that are quite frankly too boring to go into here and handles start at £15 (you can, if you wish, just buy the handle and fix it yourself if you come over all practical). If they have your handle in stock, then they can fix it the same day; if they don't they can order it from abroad (Italy or wherever) and this obviously takes a little more time. Michael's

Shoe Care, 10/12 Procter Street, London WC1V 6NX, tel: 0171 405
7436, said they would need to see it but it would cost from about a
tenner for fitting and a handle. If they don't have a match, then it's
a different quote and they can try to get one or make one . . . phew.
Handles, what a bloody nightmare, eh? Take care of yours, readers.

Always a reader on hand to help though:

With reference to John of Swansea's query about his pigskin briefcase, I had
a similar problem in replacing a calf handle on a very old French-made briefcase. I discovered a company called Mayfair Customer Service, who were
able to replicate the handle exactly to the pont of seemingly ageing the
leather. They are contactable on 0171 499 6401. – *Emma Paggini, London*
Wow, thanks, Emma. That's a good old number to know.

Can you tell me where I can buy fake fur by the metre to cover a coat collar?
Thank you. – *E. Scott, Edinburgh*
For goodness' sake, have you looked anywhere? I do think some of
you just use me as some sort of servant! Come on now. Fake fur is
sold just about anywhere and everywhere, you lazy sod. But,
because it's nearly Christmas and as I write I am munching on an
early boozy mince pie (my husband makes them far too alcoholic,
hic), I shall help you. Johnny Loulou have all sorts from tiger print
in gold, cheetah print in grey with black spots to plain black and
brown. The plainer ones start at £20 per metre, going up to £45 for
something more exotic. You have a branch in in the St James Centre, Edinburgh (0131 556 9121), so go have a look.

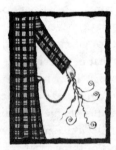

The cord of my pre-war woollen dressing gown has at last unravelled and
no sensible replacement locally available (all are too short, too thin, and
have mean tassels that snarl each other). I want something heavy, about
four yards long, with a certain dignity. – *Keith Lysons, Matlock*

Oh, Keith, replacing one's dressing-gown tassel is not easy. I can't believe someone hasn't started up a business doing this. Your best bet is to go to your local haberdashery store and buy a length of curtain cord and then a tassel. (If you need to seal off the cord to stop it unravelling you can either stitch it or glue it.) My favourite store in the world, Johnny Loulou, do a large selection that are usually used for furniture (in the haberdashery section they also have pre-made ones – the selection isn't as big as if you make your own but still go and see). Apparently they get asked this a lot: it costs from 79p a metre. You can order over the phone but you'll need to know exactly what you want. Or you could ring Jessops of Nottingham, which is your nearest Johnny Loulou branch, on 0115 941 8282 and ask for the haberdashery department. They know lots of specialists that they deal with and they might (*might*) be able to track something down for you if you tell them exactly what you want.

Tessa Dodd wrote in with a practical solution that I knew Keith would like, as he had written in before wanting to find people that made DIY moccasins kits – very hands on.

There is a solution to the problem of the deteriorated dressing-gown tassel. Anne Dyer of Westhope College runs courses in tassel-making. She is an expert in many crafts and excels in constructing these particular creations. Her excellent tuition would enable any pupil to produce tassels ranging from a delicate concoction of a few silken threads to a magnificent creation suitable for Buckingham Palace. – *Tessa Dodd, Shropshire* Contact Anne Dyer at Westhope College, Craven Arms, Shropshire SY7 9JN (01584 861293) for details on this. Sounds fab, might go meself.

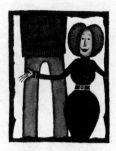

BIG . . . small
and in-betweeny sizes
of all manner of things: clothes,
shoes, maternity wear . . .

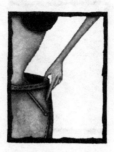

I have a real problem finding trousers to fit, so much so that I have lived in leggings for years. I have tried everywhere; not even the designer labels are any good. I have a fairly average figure (size 14), but I am hollow-backed, so that if they fit me around the hips, they are hopelessly big around the waist. I long to be able to wear smart trousers. Do you know of any designer or shop whose trousers might fit me?
– T. Baxter (Mrs), Luton

This a widespread problem, mostly because the most crucial fit in trousers – the crotch – is rarely measured. Stephen Gray, Professor of Communications and Computer Graphics at Nottingham Trent University, may be the man to change all this. He has brought a measuring booth to this country from France called the Telmat. At the Nottinghamshire International Clothing Centre in Hucknall you can have every part of you measured in 3D for £5 a time. In time he hopes that designers and stores will use his findings to reassess people's measurements (to be really futuristic, he thinks one day our measurements will be stored on smartcards and via a PC you will be able to find out what stores make clothes that fit you the best). In the meantime, have a pair made for you. I can highly recommend a couturier dressmaker called Olney Originals (01234 241440) who are not a million miles from you (they will also travel to London for meetings with their clients). They can source the fabric for you if you wish, and will make up a toile (the same garment but in calico) before they go ahead and make the item in the proper fabric. Three to four fittings ensure a perfect fit. Prices obviously vary according to the style and fabric that you choose, but as a guide a pair of simple tapered trousers in a wool-mix crêpe would cost £180. Considering how comfortable and flattering a well-fitting pair of trousers can be, this is actually very good value for money. [Others should look at the 'Dressmakers' directory at the back of the book to get the details of a dressmaker nearer home.]

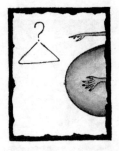

I've just found out that I am expecting my first baby. Having spent all my adult life striving for a reasonable level of style, a preliminary look at what's available in maternity wear has left me thinking that I'll have to go into solitary confinement for six months. I've been unable to find any specialists in my immediate area and should be extremely grateful if you could advise on mail-order companies or other retailers catering for mums to be.
– L. Strange, Wigan

This is a real problem for a lot of women. Who decided that pregnant women develop a penchant for large bows and polka dots? But there are some things that can make your life easier, such as maternity tights and leggings; other than that you don't need to go near a maternity shop unless you want to. OK, the sensible advice first. Blooming Marvellous are one maternity mail-order company that do a good range of basics (call 0181 391 4822 for a catalogue). They often also do a starter kit of some sort: e.g., dress, T-shirt and leggings in winter; shorts, T-shirt and vest in summer – that sort of thing. Lots of their styles are really quite simple and not bad at all. Dorothy Perkins also do maternity wear (enquiries: 0171 291 2706), as do Hennes (enquiries: 0171 255 2031), so look out for local stores. One other company, Formes, that have been going for just over three years in this country, are a cut above the rest. The clothes are designed and manufactured by Formes, so they all go together. They have three shops in London (and branches in Guildford, Manchester, Nottingham and Edinburgh). There is also a mail-order catalogue (call 0181 689 1122). Their party wear is excellent – stylish and classy, just like 'normal' party wear but for pregnant wimmin. But throughout my pregnancies I didn't wear one piece of maternity wear. Depending on what I was doing, I wore really tight Lycra T-shirts a couple of sizes bigger than I normally would with, say, one of my husband's old shirts left undone (very art-teacherish) over the top; little A-line silk slips from Fenwicks and Knickerbox; or little floral summer dresses (if poss empire line), with biker boots and my cut-off sweaters; devore shirts (Boden) over silk/satin pyjama bottoms with drawstring waists; stretch velvet dresses. I also had this shirt which I loved and as it got tighter I slit the sides to make them look like side vents, just to make it last a bit longer (it easily sewed back up again afterwards). Basically I wore whatever I wore normally, but bigger or adapted slightly. I know it's not easy – some women put weight on all over – but hopefully one of the companies/solutions I have listed will help you. Good luck.

I am 4'11" and have great difficulty finding clothes to fit me, particularly coats and jackets. I am currently looking for a raincoat, but even size 8, petite fit, is too large, in width as well as length. Where can I find smaller sizes? I am prepared to travel a reasonable distance. – *Karen, Canterbury*
It does surprise me that although things in the bigger-sizes department are still bad, clothes for the smaller women are harder yet to find. You didn't specify a price, so I have tried to trawl across the board for you: Marella, Sportmax and Max Mara (0171 287 3434 for stockists) are all part of the same family and are worth a look because their sizes come up very small. For autumn 1998, Marella have done a silver tonic belted mac in sizes 6–16, so I'd be really surprised if that doesn't fit. The closest stockist to you is Silks, 59/61 High Street, Tunbridge Wells, Kent. Burberry also do the king of raincoats, their world-famous trench-coat (double- or single-breasted), in sizes 6–14, which come in petite/regular/long and extra-long length. There is also a short mini belted version of the raincoat, again in sizes 6–14, which I think would be particularly good for you (ladies' raincoats start at £395). If size 6 is *still* to small (which is unlikely), Burberry do their classic trench in children's sizes (prices start at £235 and they are sized 2–16 years). I hesitate to suggest children's clothes as I know some petites find it insulting (even though you benefit from no VAT), but Burbie's children's trench is very classy. All of their trench-coats and raincoats come in various colours and fabrics too various to mention here; they have no stockists in Canterbury but if you call their mail-order/enquiry number on 0171 734 5929 they will be able to help you. And for those interested in other petite things, here is a quick list of people who

cover petites with enquiry numbers so you can find your nearest stockist: Bhs (0171 262 3288); Debenhams (0171 408 4444); Dorothy Perkins (0171 291 2606); Windsmoor (0181 800 8022); Wallis (0181 910 1333); Principles (0171 291 2351); Little Women (07071 780647 for a catalogue) and finally Richards (0181 910 1300). [Of course, another alternative is to look through the 'Dressmakers' directory at the back of the book and have whatever you want made to fit you perfectly.]

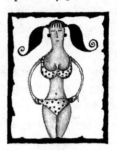

I am a fifteen-year-old schoolgirl with a bikini problem. I spent the whole of last year looking for a bikini, rather unsuccessfully. I appear to be having the same luck this year. My problem is that I am a 34c but require only size 8 bottoms. Do you know of anywhere that sells bikini separates, preferably in the West Midlands area? I would be prepared to spend up to £50.
– Naomi Geffen, West Midlands

This is such a widespread problem because you will find that people either make cupped swimwear (i.e. a 34c rather than just a catch-all 34) *or* sell tops and bottoms separately. This is all covered comprehensively in the 'Swimwear' directory at the back of the book; look in particular at Fantasie, Margaret Ann and Splash Out (who make swimwear to order).

I am blessed with a petite daughter. She is thirteen and wants to wear stylish clothes. She is about a size 6 and under 5'; her pals are blossoming above her. We can manage to find nice tops – Oasis, French Connection and other high street stuff, but we are completely stumped on trousers and skirts. The smallest Gap jeans are too big and Next size 8 is wrongly cut for her. Do you know of any good makes that we can try? I live very near Brent Cross and can get to the West End easily, but I would like to know where to look as I am limited in energy. P.S. I am a size 16 and her older sister is a size 12! This is new territory for us all.
– Lynette Craig, London

Have you tried Tammy? They are part of the Etam group and they
do up-to-the-minute fashion clothes for girls from nine to fourteen.
The clothes come in sizes according to centimetre length, your
daughter would most probably need size 152 or 158. Prices are very
reasonable indeed and they also do swimwear (Tammy's own),
which starts from £14. They have 200 shops, either stand-alone sites
or within Etam shops. Call them on 0171 636 5747 for details of
your most convenient stockist (there is one at 484 Oxford Street).
You should also have a look at Girls Unlimited, Dorothy Perkins's
young girls' range (for ages seven to fourteen), and they have a
branch in Brent Cross (in the DP store), but should you need it the
enquiry number is 0171 291 2606. Another suggestion from my
friend and petite style guru Nikki is to try a label called ICB. This is
not a cheap option, but I have included it because a) you might be
rich and b) it might be relevant to other people reading this. They
start at a UK size 4 and have fabulous trousers, but they cost around
£100; they are stocked by Harvey Nichols in Knightsbridge and Selfridges in Oxford Street. ICB's enquiry number is 0171 823 1145.
Middle price range, try French Connection Junior, which goes up to
age twelve (0171 399 7200); Jigsaw Junior goes to age twelve and the
'proper' ladies' range starts at size 8 (0171 491 4484).

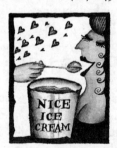

I am 5'6" and a size 18–20. The 20 comes on top as I am very busty. I am
totally bored with most clothes in larger sizes, as they either seem to
swathe you in layers of shapelessness or make you look like a hideous
bossy person working in a building society with no taste. Skirts and
trousers aren't too much of a problem, but I would love to find somewhere
that sells nice tops and jackets that would celebrate my magnificence
rather than try to make me look like a trainee nun. As I play football and
swim, I am a nice curvy shape. My partner adores me and has threatened to
tie me down and force-feed me Häagen-Dazs if I go on a diet, but is also

very interested in funding some new clothes. We regularly travel quite a bit around the UK, so distance is no object. I already enjoy spending lots of money on hats, shoes, etc. and really love nice things. Any ideas?
– *Elizabeth, Plymouth*

With all this talk of foreplay and ice-cream, HD might well sign you up to star in their next commercial. You sound like a glorious woman – my husband wants your phone number. This bigger-size business really makes me cross, I get so many letters like yours and I can tell it's a real problem not being able to find nice clothes. A reader from Bath wrote me the most brilliant letter (thank you) full of good advice, which I shall pass on; not all of it will be relevant to your problem but I am sure there are many others it will help: 'There is one absolute gem of an undies shop worth a trip from miles, Perfect Fit, 50 Temple Street, Keynsham (west of Bristol), tel: 0117 986 0950. Their bras go up to 38HH and if, like me, you need a bit of tummy support even the all-in-ones go up to 44DD. There is also Margaret Ann (01985 840520), who works from home and can get lusciously enormous undies/swimwear direct from Germany and Scandinavia, where it is not a disgrace to be buxom. Two of my favourite shops for the tall, big and bold are Base, 55 Monmouth Street, London WC2 (0171 240 8914) – they have really smart designs for large and tall business girls – and Ken Smith's Designs at 6 Charlotte Place (off Charlotte Street, London W1, tel: 0171 631 3341) – they are always so welcoming in there.' Some other readers recommend Magnum in Hants (01489 891900), which stocks sizes 16–28. [Also, of course, you must look at the 'Size 16 Plus' directory at the back of the book, which is stuffed full of fab places that stock nice clothes in sizes larger than a size 14.] Finally, on the subject of hats, have you seen Philip Treacy's sublime designs? They are breathtakingly expensive, but if you're interested call for an appointment on 0171 259 9605. He also does a much cheaper line for Debenhams.

P.S. It was this letter that prompted me to create the 'Size 16 Plus' directory, which has proved to be enormously popular. And, thanks to that reader in Bath, I discovered the truly fabulous Margaret Ann, who holds one of the coveted 'Dear Annie' gold stars [see 'Gold Stars' chapter]. And Häagen-Dazs did get in contact and sent the lovely Elizabeth lots of vouchers for free ice-cream!

I have just discovered the only place I knew I could rely on to cater for my size 9½ feet has been taken over and will not be making any summer styles to fit me! Have you any suggestions? I'm not that fussy really, as long as I can wear something. It helps if it fits, flatters and is comfortable. I've trawled around a few places for suitable men's items that aren't too gruesome or clumpy but no luck yet. – *Diana Pasek-Atkinson, Nottingham*

Thank you for the drawings of your feet, side view and top view, and all your compliments which modesty has made me edit out of your letter. I have picked your problem to publish but I have had hundreds of letters from people with the same problem so it's obviously widespread, and such is the level of research I have done into this subject that I cannot possibly print all I have found here. What I am doing is compiling a bit of a directory thing [. . . which is just what I did, and the 'Big Shoe' directory can be found at the rear of this book]. There is also a 'Footwear for Special Needs' booklet from the British Footwear Association, which costs £3 (0171 580 8687).

I have an uncle who is very tall and has real problems finding clothes to fit. Can you suggest anywhere for him to try? – *Alex, St Albans*

Oh dear. I'm not having a marvellous week this week. There has been a bit of a hitch with getting out one of my directories, due to a particularly greedy pig called Paddington who made a dreadful mess of one of my computer disks. He likes to come into the house, and being an extremely rare and expensive piggy we tend not to scold him (although I do shout bacon at him occasionally and that sends him trotting off). My eldest, Leonardo, bless him, has been trying to help me but, being only seven, seems to be more interested in spreading Nutella about my keyboard. So, Alex, this is just a taster: High and Mighty is a retail and a mail-order company for king-sized men – both tall and large (enquiries: 0800 521542). Land's End is a mail-order company which offers 'men's tall', 'men's big' and 'big and tall' sizing, as well as regular (0800 220 106). Your uncle should also try Hackett, as all their trousers (casual and formal) are unfinished so any length can be catered for (enquiries: 0171 730 3331; there are shops in London and also a mail-order catalogue). If he comes to London he can try Atlas Man's Shop, 197 Cricklewood Broadway, London NW2 3HS, tel: 0181 450 6556.

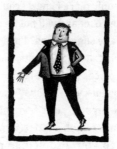

When pig control was reinstated I went on to do a 'Menswear' directory, which covers all sorts of items and can be found at the back of the book, so now Alex's uncle can have a good read through it, because he may find some 'non-specialist' places will also be able to help him.

I am a rather 'large' person (twenty stone) who would desperately like to find a tailor who has the desire to make a beautifully cut suit for someone of my size. It has been my experience that however much one pays (and money is no object), tailors just do not give as much attention to big people. I do not expect them to make me look ten stone, or want them to – I am very happy about being fat – but I would love to feel comfortable in a really good suit. I spend at least eight months in England every year and I am sure there must be a tailor somewhere who can help.
– *J. Ryan (Mr), Cashel, Co. Tipperary*

You sound like a great chappie with a sound attitude to life. And the rate I am going – with my eating due to the stress of doing this book – I shall be nigh on twenty stone quite soon myself; perhaps then we can get a discount for double orders! I am very sad that your experience is that tailors do not give as much attention to big people. From my files I have a letter from a Mr Frank Boland from Co. Kildare, who wrote in to recommend 'B. Lynch and Sons, 62 Lower Camden Street, Dublin 2, tel: 003 531 475 1642. They are a family business founded in 1932 who do very good work. Both my older brother and myself deal there.' Fabulous.

Why can't I find fasanabel cloths for my age, eight years/nine years old. Oilly is cool, but a little expensive. Laura Ashely is too babyish. I would like a long skeirt and a fited cardeycan.
– *Daisy and Chloe Price, Loxwood, West Sussex*

There are three ranges I think you should look at. First is Jigsaw, who do a splendid range for juniors from two to twelve years – very

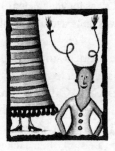

much in the spirit of their grown-up range. The main stockist for this is at 126/127 New Bond Street, London W1Y 9AF, tel: 0171 491 4484. French Connection Junior, which covers sizes 2–12, also do some great interpretations of grown-up fashion (like a couple of seasons ago they did baby Prada skirts), so call 0171 399 7200 for your nearest stockist. Another good range but perhaps too expensive for everyday wear (save up that Christmas money) is agnes b's Enfant range for girls (also boys) up to twelve years. Styles are very simple and prices are around £32 for a T-shirt (enquiries: 0171 225 3477). There is much better stock in their Paris stores than here, so should you or your parents go there, get them to stock up for you (2 rue du jour, get out at Les Halles metro). And be absolutely sure to get the mini Boden catalogue; they do some superb little things up to age twelve and as it's mail order you can peruse from the comfort of your bedroom (call 0181 453 1535 for a catalogue). The Children's Warehouse is a mail-order company for ages up to twelve; they stock basic quality clothing, plus lots of fun clothes with masses of colour (enquiries and mail order: 0181 752 1166). They also have a factory shop at Unit 4, 44 Colville Road, London W3 8BL. And just in case you have some younger brothers or sisters, two suggestions. Bobux makes soft leather shoes for babies and toddlers, in a multitude of different colours and designs. There are four sizes which cater for babies up to twenty-four months; they have no laces or Velcro but they have ankle elastic (enquiries about mail order or nearest stockist: 0181 677 9468). If you are ecologically minded young ladies, Eco ClothWORKS catalogue offers bedding and clothing, but only for the under-fives, made from organic cotton (call 0181 299 1619 for a catalogue).

One of my sons, who is twenty years old, is only 5'1" and has great difficulty finding nice clothes to fit. Is there a shop in London or elsewhere

which specializes in small sizes for young men? Harrods used to have a youth department which was quite useful, but this closed years ago.
– *David Fuegi, Colchester*

When you're next in London, go to Selfridges, who have loads that will be right. Their Kids Universe stocks Ralph Lauren Polo, Gant, Timberland, Chippie, DKNY, Calvin Klein, Moschino, Versace; size 16 in this department would probably best fit his size and they are all cool labels for a young man to wear. Also try Aquascutum in Regent Street (0171 734 6090); their jackets start at 36" chest in a shorter than regular length and they have short-fitting trousers to cater for their Japanese customers.

As an avid reader of your column in the *Independent on Sunday*, I am writing regarding an ongoing problem with the sizing of Marks & Spencer knickers. They are unfortunately sized 8–10, 12–14, 16–18, etc. As I (and my daughters) are size 10, the knickers are either too skimpy and uncomfortable (8–10) or too large and baggy (12–14). Why on earth can't they make size 10–12? I have written to M&S but received an unsatisfactory 'take it or leave it' reply. Any chance of you taking up the case? – *Susie, Swansea*

Yes, I remember the moment when I went in and saw life as we knew it had changed. Sheer pride prohibited me from buying a 12–14, yet 8–10 was too compromising. I think it was one of the biggest mistakes M&S made, forcing customers to choose between comfort and vanity. Marks & Spencer said that they changed to dual sizes in the first place because that's what the customer was saying she wanted. But now the customer is saying she wants single sizes back and good old Marks & Spencer are trialling this again, so by the time you read this we shall have our single-sized pants again (in sizes 8–22)! Ring 0171 935 4422 for details of your nearest stockist.

Clothes enable you to express personality – don't they? Help, I'm having a hard time being myself at present! Can you assist? I am 5'10" and a 12/14 with an inside-leg measurement of 34". Despite a creative and broad-minded approach to shopping, I can't find trousers to fit. All the retailers who are now doing longer lengths – M&S, Oasis, Next, etc. – aren't hitting the mark. Long Tall Sally use cheap materials and tend to design like tall means wide. So what is a girl to do? Are there any British designers/labels I've omitted from trials or should I expand my shopping horizons and go to New York to seek out unfinished 'pants', or Europe to find longer brands? Please don't be deceived into thinking I love shopping – I'm just keen to be

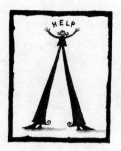

clothed as I wish. As yet I haven't won the Lottery, so my price range is not going to be in the hundreds. I do have your dressmakers list but until the ready-to-wear angle is exhausted I don't want to go down this route. One last thought: what do those super, and not so super, models do for limb-covering togs – surely not all made-to-measure? Hoping you can help.

– Sarah Morrison, south Leicestershire

Well, models wear expensive designer gear, don't they? Gucci, for one, make long, long trousers; some come unfinished, so length isn't really a problem. You would need a 42 or 44 Gucci (call them on 0171 629 2716 for your nearest stockist.) The Boden catalogue do 34" unfinished velvet jeans, two styles, £50 and £58 (call 0181 453 1535 for a catalogue). La Redoute have trousers in two and sometimes three lengths – under 5'7", between 5'7" and 5'9" and over 5'9"; Taillissime also do trousers for over 5'9" (call 0500 777 777 for a catalogue from both La Redoute and Taillissime). And lots of readers have in the past recommended Racing Green (0990 411 1111) as being very good for people with long legs and arms; they do an extra-long leg length on their trousers.

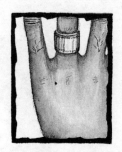

do you? i do
wedding palavas
boys and girls and weddings

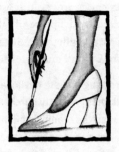

I am to be matron of honour at my sister's wedding in six months' time and am having a two-piece outfit made from turquoise blue silk – long-sleeved top with peplum and straight, mid-calf-length skirt. I am also having a matching pillbox-type hat made, but don't know what to do about the shoes, either colour or heel size. My sister, who is 4" shorter than I am, is having an old pair of flattish court shoes covered to match her outfit. While I don't want to tower over her, I think I would look better in a highish heel. Have you any suggestions? And what about colour: if they must be an exact match, then how on earth do I achieve that? Yours in desperation.
– *Sheila C. Ross, Solihull*

I would suggest you wear a bar shoe, which is like a 1920s shoe with one bar and button fastening. It is very thoughtful of you not to want to tower over her, but it sounds as if you already do! A shoe with a 2" heel will be comfortable without being ridiculous. What you might like to do is call Gamba on 0171 437 0704 (their shop, for those interested, is at 3 Garrick Street, London WC2). They do a catalogue of various styles of shoes (ballet pumps, court shoes, Louis-heeled shoes, booties) in satin which can easily be dyed with Dylon Satin Shoe Colour. Prices for the shoes start at £42.95 and go up to £110, sizes 2–8. It comes in twelve colours, costs £1.95 for a 50ml bottle and applicator and one bottle will dye up to three pairs of shoes. If you want to get an exact colour match, then you can send a swatch of your turquoise silk fabric to Dylon and they will provide you with the exact recipe of which satin shoe colours you need to combine to achieve this. The name and address to write to is Annette Stevens, Consumer Advice, Dylon International Ltd, Lower Sydenham, London SE26 5HD. Their consumer advice telephone number is 0181 663 4296. You have left plenty of time, which is good, and I hope this advice helps you achieve an exact match, which I think you need with your colour outfit. Or try Julia Taylor: she dyes shoes any colour (she mixes her own) but you need to post your shoes and a piece of fabric in the desired colour to her so she can assess whether your shoes can be dyed or not. Anyway, prices from £30; all enquiries to 0171 289 3966.

I am getting married in the spring and am having a dress made from some beautiful pale gold Thai silk that I recently purchased. I have decided that I would like to wear a veil but all the readily available white and cream ones in the shop look ridiculous when held against the fabric. I have contacted several bridal shops, both national chains and smaller independent retailers, to try to find somewhere that will make me a veil in a pale gold colour or even dye one to match the fabric, but with no success. Do you have any suggestions? Many thanks. – *Katie Mansfield, Nottingham*

Have you thought about having a veil in a fabric other than tulle? This would not only give you more scope but, from the sounds of your dress, might actually be a more suitable alternative. You could use georgette for a stiffer veil or chiffon for a softer, more drapy one. I am certain you can get both fabrics in pale gold (indeed, I have some pale gold georgette from John Lewis). If the idea appeals but you can't find the right colour, you could try dyeing it yourself; both fabrics are available in white and you can experiment with different-coloured gold dyes. I have no idea what the style of dress is, so it is difficult for me to suggest alternatives to a veil (and if you really want a veil, why compromise – it's your wedding day after all). I also suggest you contact a wonderful textile and accessory manufacturer called Nigel Atkinson, who does a lot of work with brides. I spoke to him about your problem and he said that he has a fantastic selection of fabrics from £150 a metre (I realize this is expensive but I wanted to give you the choice) and he has a dressmaker who can make it up for you. Call his office (0171 284 0316) for details of price, etc. [And don't forget to have a look in the 'Sew, Sew' chapter for a few more hints on who does fabrics.]

Next year my fiancé and I plan to marry in England. He is Indian, and a Muslim, and I am averse to wearing a meringue dress. Would you advise me where to buy something appropriate for the day? I had thought of a beautiful, fitted, embroidered salwar kameez? I am a size 16/18 top and size 14 bottom (with broad shoulders). – *Alison, Cranleigh, Surrey*

A meringue only suits raspberries, whereas a selwar kamiz (as Kiki at Ritu spells it) or sari is both beautiful and flattering to far more

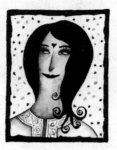

body shapes. Ritu is at 16 North Audley Street, London w1y 1we, tel: 0171 491 4600. They have hundreds of outfits and you really need to go in to see them, but to give you an idea, here is a taster, ranging in price and opulence. The *ghagra/choli* is a very traditional outfit of a chiffon skirt with long fitted blouse in brocade, with gold thread embroidery around the neck and sleeves. You wear it with a matching two-metre scarf in organza. Kiki has mentioned the beige or peach colourway in particular. The *ghagra/choli* costs £300. Or for £400 you can get an off-white selwar kamiz (tunic and loose trousers) with very traditional embroidery in gold thread, offset with soft pink and green silk thread around neck, cuffs and bottom of tunic. Trousers are drawstring with embroidery at hem and this is worn with a two-metre scarf which is also embroidered and can be worn in place of a veil. £450 will buy you a four-piece ensemble of a long tunic (kamiz), selwar, scarf in beige, with a long sleeveless coat in rust. This is styled in the tradition of the Mogul courts of India. The tunic, selwar and scarf have fine gold embroidery and the coat is in gold brocade. It sounds divine – I want one. Finally, for £650 you can have something similar to the £450 one but in off-white, with jacket in gold brocade. This has lots of work on it and is highly ornate. Even if you don't end up buying one it will give you inspiration, but my guess is you will be bewitched. Best of luck with the wedding.

I am in need of inspiration. I am getting married next year in a hot climate (Cyprus) and am trying to investigate what to wear. Are there any magazines which promote 'groomwear' as well as bridal wear? – *Peter, via e-mail*
Well, all the bridal magazines do occasionally have a token man in there, but I find their attire a little uninspiring. When my best friend got married to her husband, he had made for him a fantastic dark green velvet suit; the trousers were flared (this wasn't that

long ago) with little bells down them and that was just by a local dressmaker [if this makes you think, have a look for a local dress-makers in the 'Dressmakers' directory at the back of the book]. A few other useful hints for different-from-the-usual stuff. Favour-brook do some fabulously dandy and ornate clothes: their Nehru jackets are £380–£600, frock coats (great idea for a wedding, oh so romantic) £470–£700, waistcoats £120–£260, trousers £170–£210 and shirts £70 (call 0171 491 2337). For waistcoats try the sublime Nigel Atkinson, who makes works of art from £500 – expensive, but we are talking fancy gear (call 0171 284 0316). Tom Gilbey (0171 734 4877) has been making bespoke stuff for thirty years. His waistcoat gallery in London has been going for the last ten years and over the past two years they have started a variety of special-ized services for grooms to be. They start with a consultation to discuss the wedding – what colours might be incorporated, etc. (and they have dealt with overseas weddings before). Then you can choose from an off-the-peg service, which includes a few garments that would be suitable for overseas weddings: waistcoats cost around £130 and suits and jackets start at around £400. Or you can choose from a made-to-measure service, so lightweight fabrics could be used. They like to be a bit different – a touch of tradition, but they work with a lot of colours, not just black; prices vary enormously here, as you can imagine. The third bit they do is a hire service, which starts at around £150 for a full outfit.

Then Kaye McIntosh got in touch via e-mail to say:

Wonder if Angels Fancy Dress (the theatrical people who do all the movies) could help Peter. Don't know if they let their outfits go overseas with indi-vidual hirers, but your correspondent should check it out. I'm prejudiced in their favour – my husband went down there as a joke before our wedding (you know, 'Don't worry, darling, I'll wear something subtle like a gorilla costume' – ha ha ha, NOT) but ended up hiring the most gorgeous Regency/Darcyesque costume. Boy, did he compete for the limelight on our wedding day. Normally he's just extremely good-looking (well, I think so) but on our wedding day he was seriously . . . well, can't describe it in cold type but I'm sure you can imagine. Something to do with those tight breeches and muscular thighs, I think. Anyway, the assistants at Angels can't do enough for you. Sure they would be only too eager to help out.
– Kaye McIntosh, via e-mail

What a fabulous idea, Kaye. To take their costumes abroad, you need written permission from the management for insurance reasons (call 0171 836 5678 for further details).

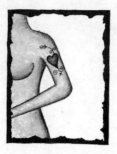

I am getting married this autumn and have a rather large tattoo on my upper arm. I am not ashamed of it, but several of my relatives have never seen it and to avoid all the explanations I'd like to wear a silver arm cuff. Where can I buy one? – *I. Prentice (Miss), London*

Two jewellery designers would be good for this and work to commissions. Jacqueline Rabun, famous for her simple silver pieces, will take about four weeks and prices start at £150; contact her on 0171 221 9820. Slim Barret, Studio 6, Shepperton House, Shepperton Road, London N1 3DF (call 0171 354 9393 for enquiries or to make an appointment), charges from £200 plus VAT for a commission. For this you will get a beautiful handmade armlet that you will want to treasure long after your wedding. Slim will work around your wedding dress design, maybe picking out the pattern or even copying the design of your tattoo, and it will take about two weeks. Ready-made styles from Slim in sterling silver start at £90. For cheaper alternatives, try the wholesale jewellers around Berwick Street, London W1.

My friend Deborah is getting married in September and has always wanted to get married wearing a Chanel suit. Unfortunately, a new one is out of the question cost-wise. Can you suggest somewhere where one could be hired or bought cheaply second-hand? The style required is the pink, to the knee, boxy-shaped one as worn by Patsy in *Ab Fab*. It also needs to be a size 16. – *Bridget Amey, Bristol*

Two places for your friend to try, neither in Bristol, though. Pandora specialize in second-hand poshness; they are at 16/22 Cheval Place, London SW7 1ES, tel: 0171 589 5289. Number Twenty, 20

High Street, Old Amersham, Bucks HP7 0DJ, tel: 01494 432043, specialize in second-hand Chanel, Armani and Dior. Obviously, stock fluctuates, so keep in regular contact.

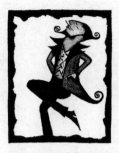

men and boys
and their problems
*men are covered throughout the book, but this
chapter looks at their very special needs*

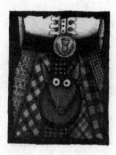

Thank heavens for your delightful, sober column. Can you please help me? Last summer I made myself a kilt using a printed fabric. However, I bumped into so many kilt snobs who told me I should have used a tartan and that I hadn't cut it right. Is there a formula for the correct way to make a kilt, and does it always have to be made from tartan? I might be a bloke, but I like to dress with a little swish and flair. And what about length? What about crushed velvet for Christmas? – *James Robinson, London*

You delightfully eccentric man. It always makes me laugh when *some* people get funny about men wearing skirts, like it is suspect or not macho. Need I remind these people that those strapping men in the Roman Empire wore skirts and in the First World War the Germans called the Highland regiments the 'Ladies from Hell' because their charges were so ferocious. Anyway, your answer, from those lovely kilt-wearing folk at the Scotch House, Highland Wear Department, 2 Brompton Road, London SW1X 7QN, tel: 0171 581 2151, is that for a traditional man's full Highland kilt, eight yards of cloth are required. The pleats all need to follow in the same direction; a kilt doesn't have to be tartan to be a kilt – the Irish Guards wear the saffron kilt, which is a self-coloured kilt made from a golden/orange cloth. Traditionally the kilt should reach just on top of the knee, give or take a few inches for individual preference. A floor-length kilt would only be worn by a woman and would be considered evening wear. So there you have the official version. I say wear your kilt any length you like (although officially it will be a skirt if it is longer than your knees) and crushed velvet for Christmastime sounds just fine to me.

What is the correct colour sock to wear with a navy suit and should I wear navy shoes to go with? And what about those thin, almost transparent socks? – *Stefano Beluovo, Edinburgh*

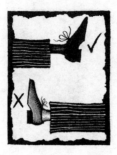

Absolutely do not wear navy shoes with a navy suit. Black shoes should be worn. As for socks, my advice is to wear navy socks, a slightly darker navy than your suit. This way the colour gradually gets darker from suit to shoe. Be sure to match the colours well – the socks should be a really dark navy. Otherwise go for black socks. As for those hideous vom-inducing thin socks you talk about . . . No. They may be all right for Julio Iglesias, but they smack of 'international playboy lifestyle'. It's like men with red cars . . . women have been taught from birth to avoid men with transparent socks. Fine-woven socks are best, understated and elegant. I am not a big fan of ribbed socks, but there is nothing really wrong with them.

What do you think of metal heel tips on shoes? – *Charles Grayson, London*
I think they are very sexy. I do like a well-turned-out man with shiny Oxford lace-ups and metal-tipped heels. That lovely clickedy-click, click as they walk down corridors, on pavements, etc. Aah. Yes, I could forgive a man like this a lot.

I am starting my first job this month and my parents have decided to invest in a suit for me. I want something that is fairly expensive as I know that you will say it is investment dressing, but what colour should I go for: grey, black or pinstripe? – *Neil Bull, London*
I can see you are a wise boy already – you know all about investment dressing and, let's face it, what better money to invest with than someone else's (you'll go far)? My advice to you is to go for none of these. Grey is nice, but it must be very, very dark grey. Light grey is not nice. Black invariably looks cheap (even if it's not) and is a bugger for picking up fluff. And personally I HATE pinstripe. I think it is naff and looks invariably cheap. Go for dark navy or charcoal, and pop along to Harvey Nichols, Selfridges, Jones in Floral Street and the Library on Brompton Road and look out for Nigel Curtiss, Yohji Yamamoto and Dries van Noten.

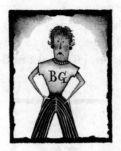

How dare you say that pinstripe looks cheap! I'll have you know that as I read your copy I am wearing pinstripe trousers! – *B.G., Canary Wharf*

Oh dear. This is my section editor, the lovely, fair, upstanding and generally supportive B.G. She was not pleased that I had said that pinstripe was cheap. But wait a minute, I was talking about *men's suits* and yes, it does make a difference, because I *do* think that pinstripe (a.k.a. chalk stripe) in men's suits is horrid. Pinstripe in other things can look rather nice. In fact, one of my favourite coats was burgundy pinstripe with a wonderful old-gold satin lining by the French designer Marcel Marongiu. I lost it one day while suffering from PMT (I get all dippy) and arrived at a party clutching my car blanket instead of my coat. I thought I had left the coat in the car, but no, it transpired that I had traipsed along Wigmore Street with the coat and the car blanket and somehow managed to drop the coat, quite without realizing it. I still miss it. So no, I don't think all pinstripe is cheap-looking and I am sure the pinstripe trousers you are wearing, dear B.G., are quite, quite magnificent. [And B.G. has now gone to edit the *Big Issue. Big Issue! Big Issue!*]

This may sound naff but what sort of men's underwear do you think is trendy? Boxer shorts? – *Francesca, Olney*

Well, I have never understood the fascination for boxer shorts, although I do admit that as a younger and more impressionable girl I too used to listen to my friends saying, 'Yeuch and he wore Y-fronts. My Dave wears boxer shorts.' To me now, wearing boxer shorts must be the male equivalent of a woman being made to wear a camisole when in fact you want to wear a nice supportive bra. I think boxer shorts are quite frankly passé. I think 'superman' pants are really cool (like briefs, really simple) and trunks (cotton jersey usually, fitted and snug over the willy-wonga area). But trunks are what I'd buy for my beloved, as his privates are as important to me as they are to him. You should also try (or your boy should) Sports Locker, 17 Floral Street, London WC2E 9DS, mail order: 0171 240 4929, who stock some well fancy stuff: Polo Sport, HOM, Björn Borg (very nice) to name but three.

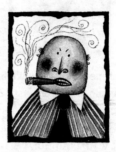

I wondered what you thought about those shirts with white collar and cuffs and coloured or striped sleeves and body. Are they smarter than plain shirts? – *Linus Harris, Kent*

Yuk is what I think about those hideous shirts with different-coloured collars. They always put me in mind of overpaid men with high blood pressure, whose nostrils invariably flare at the wrong moment. To my mind *nothing* is more stylish than a crisp white or blue shirt. If my husband ever went out to work wearing one of those different collar and cuff coloured shirts he'd be coming home to a different house (baby, I'm joking).

I'm in a spot of bother. I cannot think what would be a suitable item of clothing to buy my girlfriend for St Valentine's Day. I don't want to be clichéd and buy lingerie . . . but I know she would like it. Where should I go for something fashionable? P.S. I have a small worry concerning cufflinks. Does one wear silk cufflinks only for evening dress and heavy cufflinks only for daywear, or does it not matter? – *J., Maidstone*

Well, lingerie is clichéd, but it is lovely to receive. Where men invariably go wrong is buying something in red and black (or all red), when few women would choose to wear scarlet underwear. You can buy something from La Perla (the Rolls-Royce of underwear as far as I am concerned) that is luxurious and she might never choose to buy for herself but would nevertheless love to wear. Also avoid 'fantasy' underwear that men buy for their women to wear but which is usually for themselves (if you see what I mean). Of course, there are some girls who like wearing scratchy lace crotchless panties or cut-out bras, but they are in the minority. What about something from Prada's new lingerie boutique in Harrods? Prices start at £45 for a pair of pants and not only is it very nice, it's also very bloody 'in'. [And you may wish to peruse the 'Underwear' directory at the back.]

Being a bit thin on top, I find I need a hat in cold weather. I have a nice red woolly one, knitted by my aunty, which I wear while walking. But I don't think it's quite right for work. What would you suggest?
– Keith, Portsmouth
Well, what work could you possibly do that a red woolly hat would not be suitable for? I think it sounds splendid and, anyway, you could always take it off just before you get into the office. Men are very bad at keeping warm, thinking it is unmanly, but given the choice between a nice, warm, glowy man and a shrivelled, cold one I know which I'd prefer.

Where can I buy a really nice purple tie? I like 'labels' but find Versace way too vulgar. – *Mr N. Timmy, Clacton-on-Sea*
Connolly (0171 235 3883), the fabulous people that make the leather interiors of my beloved Aston Martins, also do fashion things. Apart from having the best, and I mean *the best*, cashmere scarves and shawls, they do knitted silk ties for £54 and, yes, they do one in purple with teeny-tiny spots in grey or yellow (very nice, I assure you).

I've been looking for a man's ring in Manchester, but they all seem the same, either sovereign, onyx, diamonds or some other old-fashioned and unimaginative design. Perhaps you know of a jeweller's that offers something original. I realize designer jewellery would be much more expensive, but, after all, it's something I will have for a lifetime. I would be willing to try anywhere in the country. Maybe you can give me some addresses.
– C. Lambert (Mr), Manchester
I certainly can. I wish I knew somewhere in Manchester. I don't, but if you come down to London visit a shop called Jess James, run by the boyishly handsome Jess Canty [see 'Gold Stars' chapter, they hold one]. It's at 3 Newburgh Street, London wiv ilh, tel: 0171 437 0199, and they stock loads of lovely stuff. Names to look for generally are Detail (0171 730 8488); Dower and Hall (0171 589 8474); Sian Evans (0171 251 6881); Diana Porter (0117 941 4953); and Jacqueline Rabun (0171 221 9820). Around the corner from Jess James, at 10 Ganton Street, London wiv ild,

tel: 0171 439 9357, is a shop called the Great Frog, much
favoured by rockers and bikers. The Lesley Craze Gallery (0171
608 0393) also stock some very unusual rings by contemporary
designers. It is, of course, worth giving all the people quoted a
ring (ha ha) to see if they have stockists closer to home. So there
you are – not many addresses as such, but lots of phone numbers
and ideas.

**I need a few crisp white shirts and maybe the odd cream or pale blue one. I
hate shopping and hope to buy a batch of shirts that will stay looking gorgeous for a long time. In the past I've had problems finding shirts that fit
well because a) all cotton shirts shrink, but not all by the same amount, b)
shops won't let you try on before you buy and c) many shops don't do different sleeve lengths. I'm forty-five, slim and tall and spend most of my
working day in shirt and tie with no jacket. I don't mind paying for quality
but have no interest in labels for their own sake. Altogether I'm bewildered
by the choice and hope you can help by guiding me to something really
stylish. – David, London**

Well, my personal favourites are from agnès b. They do a classic
one-pocket shirt for men (and a similar style for women). They
don't come in different arm-lengths, but for me it is the defini-
tive shirt. Why? Well, the 'handle' of the shirt is exceptional, due
to the weight of the cotton used (it's meaty), its styling is simple
and it wears well, although it is not the most formal of shirts so
may not be right for everyone. They come in white or pale blue,
cost £72 and are available from the branches in Westbourne
Grove, Hampstead Heath Road and Floral Street (call 0171 379
1992 for further information). They will certainly let you try on
before you buy. I am also rather confused that your shirts
shrink: because mine never do, even though I put my cotton ones
in at a boil wash. What do you do with them? (And I mean that
kindly.)

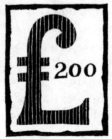

I am starting a new job soon that will involve wearing a suit. I am looking for something conventional but not too 'stuffy'. Of course, having just graduated I am broke, but if you think I should spend more that the couple of hundred quid I was thinking of I can ask my parents for a sub. Do you have any advice? – *George Stewart, Surrey*

You can pick up an excellent suit from Jigsaw or Marks & Spencer for a couple of hundred quid. There really is no need to spend more at this stage. As the new boy, you will only inspire envy and suspicion if you turn up in an £800 + suit.

Reading your column is far more fun than going shopping, which is my least favourite activity. Please could you spare a thought for the likes of me (I can't be the only one). I really like clothes that are stylish and fit well, and don't mind spending what it costs – but have almost no time to go and buy them. When I try it is often a disaster because I've no idea where to look, or indeed what to look for. My last splurge was about ten years ago, and as all those clothes are falling apart I now need pretty well everything: a dinner suit, a couple of summer-weight suits, ditto for winter, a few jackets, several pairs of shoes – the works, in fact. My ideal would be to get the lot in one day, then thankfully forget about clothes buying for several more years. A friend in New York tells me they have 'shopping consultants' who will advise both on where to go and what to get. I wonder if this service exists over here? I am regretfully assuming you yourself are not available. (Though if you were you could make a fortune – if Samantha Fox charges £10,000 to attend a party you could charge the earth!) Alternatively, how about made to measure? – *David, London*

Oh, David, it's you again. [I think you appear in this book more than anyone else.] You sound quite rich. Are you also good-looking? In which case maybe I could make myself available (for shopping only, of course). But no, p'raps best left. For now. Anyway, shopping consultants do exist here and most stores have them; it is a service few of us make use of. For you I have concentrated on shops that I think would suit you, but generally most stores will provide this if you ask. Selfridges in Oxford Street, London W1, provide a personal shopping service which is on an appointment basis and is 'one to one'. It can be arranged during opening hours, Mon–Wed, 10 a.m.–7 p.m., Thurs, Fri, 10 a.m.–8 p.m., Sat, 9.30 a.m.–7 p.m. and Sun, 12 a.m.–6 p.m., and they need about a week's notice (call 0171 318 3536 or fax 0171 318 3300). The service is free, there is no obligation to buy and no minimum spend. You are also encouraged to bring in your own clothes if you just want to finish off your look with a jacket or whatever. Jones in Floral Street, tel: 0171 240 8312, sell some wonderful, slightly more unusual clothes from various designers. They have a client book and all the sales staff have their 'own' customers whom they'll ring once they get to know their tastes, and tell them if something's come in they think they'll like. Harvey Nichols in Knightsbridge also provide this service and it is also free and available during store hours. There is usually a week's waiting list. To book an appointment call 0171 235 5000. Browns of South Molton Street also provide this service free and it is available at all times, including after opening hours if necessary (10 a.m.–6 p.m., Mon–Sat; 10 a.m.–7 p.m., Thurs). Their service is very flexible and includes local deliveries to homes and hotels (for which you will have to pay extra). They have a VIP room for extra privacy. There is no waiting list and the men's shop can be contacted for an appointment on 0171 514 0038. So you see, David, you don't really need me. Shucks.

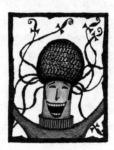

My father is seventy-five years old, lives in Australia and has a sense of humour. He recently wrote that he is 'getting thinner on top', and as I know that he has always been reluctant to visit the barber, I would love to buy him a baseball cap with a long, grey ponytail attached to it. Do you know if anyone in London sells them? – *Christine, London*
I have tried all the usual joke/party/toy shops for you and they didn't have any, although one kind chap told me that you can sometimes get them in some of those little shops in Carnaby Street or Covent Garden (the sort that also sell policemen's helmets, you know). Why don't you make him one? The haberdashery sections of big department stores sometimes do fake hair bits for puffing out buns and the like, and then you can just pin it on. This seems the best and cheapest way to put a smile on your father's face. (If

you're not funny about these things you could even ask your hair-dresser to keep a clean, shorn length of hair for you, although I think you'll have more luck if you don't hold out for grey.) However, if you are really serious then in the wig department of Selfridges they do fake ponytails for £37 (Oxford Street, London w1, tel: 0171 629 1234), or Trendco (229 Kensington Church Street, London w11, tel: 0171 221 2646) do them for £49. This does seem rather excessive, not to say expensive, but I try to leave no stone unturned.

And here's David again:

I have just been reading your column and was intrigued by the note from Christine (asking for a baseball hat with ponytail attached). I have just been on holiday in Oz and came upon a highly unusual pharmacy in Noosa Heads, Queensland. This pharmacy sells more hats than drugs, and I bought the most unbelievably hilarious tea-cosy hat which has long, thick black plaits attached which dangle from the back (one size only); it is very loosely elastic, which means it fits my enormous head beautifully, but it looks equally good on my six-year-old nephew. I have just called them (Noosa Heads Pharmacy, tel: 006 175 474 9733, fax: 006 175 447 3298). They will send one anywhere in Australia for the price of A$27.99 plus a very reasonable A$5 p&p. I didn't think to ask if they do baseball hats with grey ponytails, but it wouldn't surprise me if they do. I have photos of the hat worn by myself and also the six-year-old. If Christine is interested, I would be happy to send them directly or via you. What a hoot if this happens! I can assure you, the hat really is GROOVY and has caused normally staid reserved people to collapse with mirth. P.S. Thank you for your very full reply to my query about shopping consultants. I will certainly take a deep breath and go for one or more of the places you mention. However, what I had in mind was a day out with an independent adviser who would start by looking me up and down (and also take a look at my existing wardrobe), instantly know what was needed and which shops to go to, then leap into the minicab I'd hired for the day, zoom round the shops with me and collect a cheque from me, leaving me kitted out for several years. I'm not specially rich but would rather spend a few thousand every ten years than a hundred or two every month, which many teenagers seem to manage and which averages out at more smackers per year than me. The adviser's fee would be well worth it, but do such exist?
– David Gardner, London w6

Dear David, you are such a regular, faithful reader that I had to reproduce your letter in its entirety. I thought it would make people laugh before Christmas. Have you been at the sherry a bit early? Thank you for the tip about the hat. I am sure that anyone in Australia who is looking for such a hat can now glide peacefully into the millennium. And yes, independent shopping advisers do exist but I don't know of any that I'd care to recommend. P.S. David, you know that I would come and look you up and down myself, but feel it would be imprudent as my beloved is away at the moment.

My delight at the renaissance of the gents' three-button jacket has speedily turned to irritation and angst . . . I stayed faithful to the style even when it languished in the doldrums but always understood that the middle button *only* was to be fastened. Now every trendy presenter on the telly is going for the full house of all three. I'm convinced that this is vulgarism on a grand scale – the very fauxest of faux pas. Your thoughts . . .?
– *Tom Gallagher, London* SE7

I called Carlo Brandelli, super-stylish freelance fashion and design consultant – he is a bit of a know-all in the 'correct' way of men's dressing – and he said, 'It is correct to have the middle button fastened at all times. You can have the top and middle buttons fastened if you are feeling sporty and have the jacket completely unbuttoned if you are wearing a waistcoat. Under no circumstances should you have all three buttons fastened as far as style is concerned. What do TV presenters know anyway?' And, yes, I do agree with him.

I recently spotted a guy wearing a button-down-collar shirt, but the collar was not the familiar 'pointy' style, but was actually rounded. I've gone around every menswear shop I can think of in central London, but have had no joy finding a shirt like this. Any clues? – *Mark Baxter, London* SE5
Interesting that you want this funky-shaped collar, and you have inspired me to buy some too, for Mr Annie. Ben Sherman have the Penny Round button-down-collar shirt, which costs £49.99. In linen/polynosic [like modal, see 'Encyclopedia'], they come in red, aqua and royal blue and are available from Debenhams branches. Call 0800 592549 for other stockists.

I have had great difficulty trying to obtain a pair of lace-up black plimsoles. They seem to have been driven out of the shops by trainers and deck shoes. I want them in an adult size 11 or 12. Can you help?
– *Dr Alex Scott Samuel, Liverpool*

A doctor! Well, I am privileged. While I have you, Dr Scott Samuel, I've had this recurring pain . . . nah, Doc, only joking. How fondly I now remember those plimmies that I used to wear at school. But how I used to hate them at the time. You are right, they are nowhere. The shops are full of hideous trainers so big and chunky one would feel compelled to have a lifestyle to fit in with them. Some places/makes do these styles but either in just children's sizes or women's. Springcourt, sold in the Natural Shoe Store in London's Neal Street, do exactly what you're looking for, but only up to a size 10. Can I throw this out to tender? Can anybody out there help Dr Scott Samuel? Waste no time in writing in.

Please tell Dr Alex Scott Samuel that black lace-up plimsoles are readily available in Zimbabwe for Z$70.00 per pair (about £3.50).
– Noreena Elwell, Harare, Zimbabwe

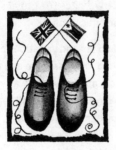

Zimbabwe has always been one of my most favourite words, ever since Angela Rippon pronounced it so emphatically while reading the news. The only thing for Dr Scott Samuel is that although the plimmies may cost £3.50, the airfare over to Zimbabwe might make it slightly prohibitive, especially with what doctors earn nowadays. Anyone popping over to Zimbabwe, buy Dr SS a pair in black, size 11 or 12. *Zimbabwe.*

And guess what? Someone did! Gai Ellis of Cambridge went to Zimbabwe and bought dear Dr Alex Scott Samuel some black plimmies. Kind or what? Dr SS was suitably grateful and Gai's place in heaven was assured.

Re your article about 'plimmies', our chain of shops can still supply the black lace-ups up to size 11 (not 12s!). We used to bring them into the country in wooden crates back in the 1950s by the 1,000s. As you say, trainers have now taken over but we can still supply at approx £3.99. P.S. We used to sell them at 9^1/2d. *– Tim Baldock, E. Baldock & Sons Ltd, 1–3 Swan*

Street, West Malling, Kent ME19 6LD, *tel: 01732 845292*

Thank you, Timmy. Your shop sounds fab. And hope that helps you when the South African ones give in, Dr Scott Samuel. Now then, about my recurring trouble . . .

I am thirty-five, a photographer and I love fly-fishing, the opera, William Morris, Pre-Raphaelite art and Triumph Heralds, of which I have two, one light blue and one dark blue. I like to dress in jeans, T-shirts, that kind of thing, and sometimes even velvet suits. My problem is that I cannot find, anywhere, black leather gloves in a size 8^1/$_2$ – 8, yes, or even 9, but not 8^1/$_2$. Please can you help me as my hands are getting cold. – *Pete, London*

Young man, where exactly have you looked? I bet you just popped into Johnny Loulou, couldn't find what you were looking for and thought, 'I'll write to that bird in the paper and let her do the work while I get pop off to do some fishing.' Visit Harrods or Selfridges. Thumb through the Yellow Pages for glove shops. Or just buy the gloves in a size nine. Goodness' sake.

Once cloth caps came in all styles and variations of styles, but from about the time Mark Phillips married Princess Anne and was seen frequently wearing a distinctive style of cap, one which was very deep at the back, the hat manufacturers seem to have abandoned all caps other than that type (except for the type cut into segments like a cake, with a button on top). Up until about five years ago I could buy a Harris tweed cap which had a depth of 3" at the back. But now all I can find are caps which are about 4" or even 5" at the back, a style I cannot wear. Can you help? – *Frank, Durham City*

James Lock, 6 St James's Street, London SW1A 1EF, tel: 0171 930 8874/5849 and mail order, have been traditional hatmakers for 300 years. They made the first bowler hat in the 1850s. They make two types of 'mean' fitting caps (what I believe you are looking for), the Glen at £45 and the Gill at £59. Kangol make the Kangol 504, which costs £20–£30, comes in tweed or plain wool and may also find favour with you (apparently this shape is becoming very fashionable again – half a million were made last year, hurrah!). It is available at House of Fraser stores and, near Durham, at Metro Centre, Gateshead, and at Anetson Clothing, Chester-le-Street. Also try Barbour Gala Forest caps, which come in sizes 6^1/$_2$ to 7^3/$_4$ and cost about £23. Call 0800 009988 for stockist enquiries, but nearest to you are Thomas Owen and Sons, 40–46 The Side, Newcastle, and 23 Fore Street, Hexham. A tip to make any woollen (unlined) cap or beret fit better is to wet it and then put it on, but as this can give you a frightful cold do it only if you are barking!

For the last fourteen years I have been addicted to black pointed shoes. I used to buy them from a shop in Oxford Street called Shelly's but about three years ago they stopped selling them. They said there was no longer a market for them. I bought the last six pairs in my size – four in leather and two in suede. But now they are all gone. My wife and I must have checked every shoe shop in London but could not find anywhere that sold pointed shoes. In desperation I called Shelly's mail-order service. They searched their database and found they still had two pairs left – one in their shop in Carlisle and another, a size too small, in Leeds. These could be the last two pairs of pointed shoes I ever have. I bought them both. Now the last pair in my size has worn out. Ahead of me I have either days crippled in pointed shoes too small to wear or a life without pointed shoes at all! Please, please, please tell me were I can find some more black, suede, pointed shoes. – *Danny Bakhshi, Harrow*

Well, Shelly's (0181 450 0066) tell me that they still stock these shoes, in black leather and black suede, but they are slip-ons with elastic at the side (maybe you wanted lace-up, you didn't say). But anyway, the leather ones come in sizes 3–11, £32.99 (style no. 37023 if you need it), and the suede ones in sizes 6–12 at £29.99 (style no. 37001). Schuh (0181 667 0320) do a black leather or suede Chelsea boot with pointy toes and a block heel, if that takes your fancy. And Ad Hoc, 4 Lancer Square, 28 Kensington Church Street, London w8 4EP, tel: 0171 376 1121, have black leather pointed flat boots with zip or elastic for £65, sizes 8–12. So mop up those tears, Danny.

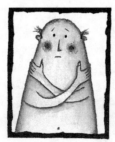

As a side effect of medical treatment for prostate cancer, I have developed breasts, which my wife tells me are a 48C cup. She suggests I wear a bra for support, but I don't want one that makes them more pronounced, for obvious reasons. Any ideas on what type and where I can get a couple. It is obviously awkward for me. – *A. Hunter, Middlesex*

You poor thing, but there is no need to be embarrassed or feel awkward. Call up the divine Margaret Ann (01985 840520), who deals with all sorts of 'sensitive' underwear problems and so is well used to being a) discreet and b) sympathetic and helpful. Off the cuff, she said she would most probably recommend a seamless sports bra from Anita (£25), as it would offer support but not exaggerate your breasts.

What's a boy to do? Girls can carry handbags, and suits can wear a jacket or carry a briefcase, but since the outlawing of bumbags as an acceptable accessory, what are we blokes supposed to do with our bits – wallet, change, keys, mobile, Newtons, A–Zs, etc.? Have you any idea on stylish and politically acceptable 'bags to be carried by hand' for men?
– Guy Marriage, London

Well, Guy, European men have for years been carrying round with them those small bags with wrist straps that are becoming increasingly popular here. YMC do 'gentlemen's purses', which are sold at Brown's Focus in South Molton Street or Duffer of St George in Covent Garden; they cost £15. Ck by Calvin Klein do a really nice Filofax-sized wallet in mottled black or brown leather. It is hand-held and would fit keys and money in, but only a tiny, tiny phone, and costs £72 (enquiries: 0171 491 9696). But any department store will sell those little bags with wrist straps. Go look.

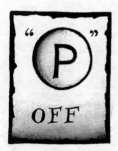

that told you
short shrift for silliness
*for those that really should
have known better*

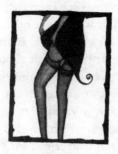

My wife always wears pop sox, which I hate. I think they're so unsexy. When we first started going out she always wore stockings and suspenders, but she won't now, saying they're uncomfortable. Will you tell her that stockings are really fashionable and that pop sox are really untrendy? – *D. Wallis, London*

Well, three guesses what the correct response to your pathetic letter is? 1. Mrs Wallis: pop sox are really untrendy and stockings and suspenders are really in, so be trendy and get yourself tackled up. 2. Why don't you compromise and she can wear hold-ups? 3. You are a stupid, stupid man with no idea. You yourself have most probably become very unsexy and you smell and your wife cannot be bothered to wear what *you* find sexy but she most probably finds uncomfortable. She most probably does all the housework, works full-time and cooks wholesome, interesting meals for you and your fifteen children. You expect her to do this wearing stockings? True, some women love wearing 'the gear' for themselves. But some don't. Feminism is about choice and your wife has chosen knee-hose. Grow up and get sexy yourself, before your wife finds herself a lover and starts wearing stockings again because she wants to.

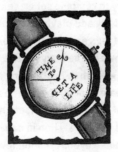

I am in dispute with my friend as to what the best watch to have is, she says Rolex and I say Cartier. Who is right? – *Simone Frasier, London*

Best? What do you mean by best? They are both brilliant watches and won't give you a moment's trouble other than possibly inspiring muscly men to cut your wrists off at traffic lights. If you and your friend have nothing better to argue about, then perhaps a spell in a soup kitchen might give you both something to think about. Of course, if you want to know what's really super-in, then the answer is a black plastic Casio watch from Argos for £20. It's water-resistant to 200 metres, which, divided by 200, should just about be level with you and your friend's IQ (combined).

I have a pretty good figure with a touch of cellulite on my upper thighs. I am going on holiday with some new friends to the Virgin Islands and I am keen to impress. I'd like to know about some good expensive swimsuits that have one of those little skirts attached that would disguise this.
– Kathryn Hart, Hampshire

I'm not sure what you seriously expect me to advise you. Chanel/Ralph Lauren/Donna Karan have done some fantastic swimsuits that will spare your embarrassment? Maybe they have, but you have a pretty good figure and a bit of cellulite. Sod it and show it off. Do you really care? Do your friends really care? Remember that starving people do not have the *luxury* of cellulite. Cellulite is due to too much good living and not enough exercise and I don't give a toning-table toss who says otherwise. Donate your holiday to a good cause, get off your butt and get it moving. But I doubt you'll do any of these. So why not stick £50 notes over the offending area. That way people will know you are filthy rich and will be too bothered being your new best friends to notice a bit of podge.

My girlfriend has the ability to combine sober, sensible clothes with something a bit more frivolous, frilly and playful without looking tasteless or overdressed. She has great legs and prefers to wear stockings when the hem length of her skirt allows it. I've bought her a white skirt and want to buy her some stockings to go with it. I'm thinking of some with a swirly lace pattern or a glittery seam or anything that has a bit of life to it. Fishnet stockings come to mind but there's always something a bit cheesy about them to my mind. I find the hosiery section in department stores a bit daunting with (to the untrained eye!) row upon row of basically the same colours made by different firms. Can you help me with any suggestions as well as the names of manufacturers so at least I'm armed when I next visit

a department store. If the answer lies in a specialist shop in London please
mention that as I visit London fairly regularly. – *Martin Forrester, Chorlton*

My dear boy. I know that some people feel that ladies and gentlemen of the press can have too much power, expressing, as they
do, feelings and opinions that may influence many. But if I
achieve one thing through this column it will be the eradication of
swirly lace tights. They are foul things that should be foisted
upon only the most unfortunate of women, perhaps as a punish-
ment for adultery, in countries that still punish for such things. If
you love your girlfriend – nay, boy, even if you *like* her, do not, I
beg you, buy her novelty tights. Words like frivolous, playful and
frilly may come to your mind, but words such as naff, passé and
Molly Ringwald in *Pretty in Pink* are the only words that come to
mine. Forgive me this violent opinion and let us get on with guiding you around the hosiery world. The best specialist shop for
hosiery in London, in my opinion, is Fogal. But they are expensive. There is a branch at 36 New Bond Street, London W1Y 9HD,
tel: 0171 493 0900, and they have a brilliant array of tights, from
boring but excellent opaques and sheers to something a bit more
'novelty'. Then you might want to pop into Fenwick, just up the
road at 63 New Bond Street (0171 629 9161), and then John Lewis
and Selfridges on Oxford Street. The brands to look for are
Jonathan Aston, as they are well known for more fancy hosiery
(in fact they have a red lacy pair if you really want), and Wolford,
for something unusual such as their seamless tights (Fatal), and,
yes, they do netty/lacy tights. You are sure to find something
among all that lot.

*Note: The following season, fancy, lacy tights became the height of fashion,
so I guess that told me.*

I have hair that hangs lank. I achieve height and curl with an electric brush,
then add lacquer to keep the style up. But any hat or headscarf, once on,
depresses all the height and I emerge utterly flattened when I take it off.
Any suggestions? – *Mrs Le Cornu, Jersey*

Well, nothing would keep your hair bouffed if you put something
on it. It's like asking a soufflé to stay souffléd if you rest a dinner
plate on it. Lummy, love, I wish I could suggest some magic Annie
trick but I can't. There are only two solutions: don't wear anything
on your head or adopt a flatter hairstyle.

I long to see my wife in a thong. I have bought her a few, but she complains that none of them is comfortable. Can you suggest one that is? Also, what is the difference between a thong and a G-string? – *Simon, Southampton*

There is no difference between a thong, G-string, or string-back pant, as they are also called. They *are* uncomfortable, although some women do like them and they have their place (brilliant for banishing VPL). But if your wife doesn't like wearing one, then that must be her choice. You try wearing one, sunbeam, and then you'll see why your wife doesn't want to.

I write to complain about your smarty-pants put-down reply to poor Simon of Southampton who longs to see his wife in a thong. I agree that thongs are not super-comfy, but aren't they mostly designed to be enjoyed while taking them off? I suggest that a useful alternative, which is comfortable and can be yanked up to look the part, are M&S lace-edged, very high-cut knickers . . . – *T.S., Newcastle*

Oh, for goodness' sake, thongs 'mostly designed to be enjoyed while taking them off'! Just what do you think this is? This is a column about FASHION problems. Simon of Southampton's wife doesn't like wearing thongs and that's that. I would have given the same sort of answer (and in the past I have) if a woman had asked me to recommend a more comfortable pair of boxer shorts if her husband didn't like wearing them in the first place. So there.

I have a boyfriend who has appalling dress sense. His actual choice of garment isn't bad, but because of his line of work he gets quite a lot of 'promotional' stuff: logoed baseball jackets advertising some new film, that sort of thing. You seem level-headed and rational. How can I get him to wear normal clothes without hurting his feelings? – *Catherine, Godalming*

Gosh, it sounds like you are going out with the modern equivalent of a sandwich-board advertising man. I could advise you to go shopping with him, leave copies of *L'Uomo Vogue* lying around, that sort of thing. But I shan't. Try this: 'You're really nice but your dress sense is misguided and it upsets me so much that I have written to a national newspaper for advice. I cannot see past the clothes you wear, so please do something about it and fast.' You sound like a woman of hidden shallows, Catherine. So let's not be too deep about it.

Do you know of anyone who makes cream-coloured ovens apart from stoves. We have ordered all other electrical items for the kitchen from

Hotpoint in linen/calico, but cannot find an oven to match. Please help.
– *P. O'Donnelly, Essex*

I had to print this because I have been getting more and more queries of a non-fashion nature. One gentleman even asked what golf clubs I recommended. I don't really mind, although very often I haven't a clue. Like in this case. I mean, I could do loads of research into it, but I fear this may be opening the flood gates. If anyone has an idea, write in to me. One question though, P. O'Donnelly. If you've ordered all your electrical bits and bobs in linen/calico, how will they stand up on their own? Ha ha ha ha.

I love your column and look forward to reading it every week. I should be delighted if you know of anyone in the UK who has imported an American computer program that gives a printout of the sizes and shapes to wear when you send in your exact measurements. It sounds wonderful and I long to have it here. I do hope you can help. I simply cannot think of where else to look! – *Sheila, London*

Sheila, my love, I am in the advanced stages of my fifth pregnancy and I haven't a clue what you're talking about. My only concern at the moment is how to get my pants up and down without having to enlist help. I have never heard of such a thing.

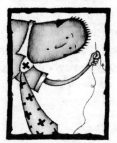

I am a consultant working in Accident and Emergency medicine. As such, I have to appear smart, yet my medical practice can involve blood splashes and other body fluids. I detest suits, especially jackets, and work in a fairly warm environment. I tend to wear M&S black trousers and cheap, white, short-sleeve shirts and tie. I would be happy to lose the tie, but it is expected of me. It can get in the way when I'm stitching. Could you suggest a smart yet practical and washable solution to my problem. Operating theatre 'greens' as in *ER* are not available.
– *Dr Please-don't-use-my-name, via e-mail*

Hello, everybody. Thank you for all your cards and good wishes.

I was keen to get back into the swing of things as soon as possible and am fortunate that I am able to work from home, although it will be a few weeks before I am fully up to speed again. Anyway, when you've done this as many times as I have, it's no big deal. Plus, my husband is showing off and dandling the new baby (who is very pretty and has black hair like him) while I get on with urgent fashion problems – although who he thinks is going to feed the pigs, I don't know. Short of wearing an apron or overalls, Doc, the like of which we see on car mechanics or Formula One racing drivers, I see no solution to your problem. Get a tie-clip and wear your normal clobber. And isn't everything washable these days?

But, of course, one of my regular and favourite correspondents, David Bonkers Gardner from London, had a reply:

Your casualty doc sounds hopeless. I've worked in several casualty departments [OK, David, no need to show off] – disposable plastic aprons are standard and invariably worn for messy tasks. If he disdains this, there's always the bow tie. This is favoured by obstetricians/gynaecologists NOT because they fancy themselves like mad BUT because they're always having to bend forward to examine pregnant tums or other things [they're called vaginas, David, tut] that prefer not to be tickled by a standard tie, thank you. Or he can tuck his tie into his shirt (as I do in my children's clinic, where the chief hazard is getting piddled on by six-week-old babes). Bless you too, David, but you never mentioned you were a doctor before. I'd have been *much* nicer to you! I do like doctors, you're all so big and so mean and so strong . . .

And David had an answer to that:

I'm honoured to be appearing in lights again in your column. Bonkers, eh? OK as long as you don't call me Bonk for short. Thank you for the helpful prompt on the technical terms employed by the – er – bits down there. I hesitate to disagree with a lady who has had five children, but as one who used to lecture in anatomy to fledgling naughty-bit doctors, may I give you the more conventional wisdom, which is that the sensitive outside part (which needs protecting from ties) is commonly called the vulva. The vagina is altogether more private and out of the way.
Really! I'll have no more of that talk on a Sunday morning, David. You really are a dreadful show-off.

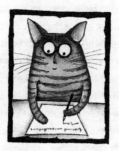

Meows, dear Annie! You may be wondering why a cat is writing to you, but I do enjoy your column each week. My humans think I'm just washing myself while I sit on the paper and stop them from reading it, but really I'm taking in every word! Anyway, I'm the cause of one of their problems and I wonder if you could help. Since humans don't have thick fur coats like me, they have to wear woollen suits and coats to keep themselves warm, and the trouble is my fur clings to their clothes (along with other threads and dog hair) and is very difficult for them to remove. The worst colours affected are navy blue and black, although red and green also seem to attract hair and my fur, and also miscellaneous 'bits'. Please do you have any suggestions as to how my humans can remove fur and other clinging items from their clothes? They have tried Sellotape (effective, but fiddly and time-consuming), a clothes brush (no use at all) and a rubber glove (this seems to be the best yet), and also storing their clothes in protective covers, but still the fur sticks! If you could find a solution, I would be most grateful, and so would my humans. By the way, my humans live in Exeter in Devon. Purrs . . . – *Otis Baker, via e-mail*

Well, Otis, your humans seem to have tried everything I would have suggested. But you seem like a nice cat, so if you really, really want to be of help to your humans and stop your no doubt cuddly fur sticking to their clothes, then I'd go out and get myself lost if I were you.

This prompted lots of people to write in, but the funniest by far was the following:

As a regular reader of your column, along with my mum, I was rather distressed by your curt treatment of Otis Baker regarding the 'fur on clothes' problem. We cats have to endure this affliction, and it can cause us distress when we are not cuddled by our parents because they are wearing dark clothes. It's a wonder that more of us don't end up seriously disturbed. As everyone around me understands, I have an opinion on – and know – everything, so of course I have the answer to the problem. Lakeland Ltd (015394 88100)make a product called Sticki-Mitts, ref. 8945, £1.95 for twenty. They are wonderful and my parents use them all the time. The clothes roller, ref. 8913, £6.95, is good too and I have seen these at Johnny Loulou, which is also my mum's favourite shop! As a finely marked tortoiseshell, I am excited by the lilac and lime-green colours that I see around for the spring and summer, as they will suit me much more than all those 'cat' prints. Incidentally, in my opinion Mum spent rather too long reading the article on men's pants today in the *Independent on Sunday*'s fashion pages. She is a teacher of more than fifty and should be past all 'that'. Ralph, my brother, now wants a pair of the Hugo Boss ones. – *Katie Austoni, Huntingdon*

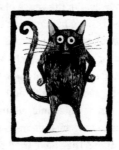

Hilarious. Loads of people wrote in to recommend the same. And I thoroughly recommend Lakeland Ltd; they make lovely, useful products and are so helpful. One final note: Lottie, an e-mail correspondent, wrote in to suggest using those green scouring pads; used dry apparently they pick up cat hairs like magic (but don't get confused and use it later for washing up – that would be disgusting).

Annie, sweetie. I think you have a wonderful job, darling, going out shopping with other people's money and having babies occasionally. The rest of us wage slaves can only writhe in green-eyed jealousy. Anyway, I am after something cheap and cheerful which has now died a death and been downsized to dusting. It is a soft T-shirt-material, off-the-shoulder top with three-quarter-length sleeves and has a knitted welt on the bottom and around the top. I know it sounds naff but I wore it with jeans or jazzed it up with skirt and heels and managed to score nearly every time I went out in it, so it's part of my men-slaying wardrobe. It was so versatile and I feel that I can never go out again if I don't get a replacement for it! I don't mind long sleeves but I would like black. I paid about £15 for it in a cheap little boutique, but despite extensive searches since – nothing. Money around

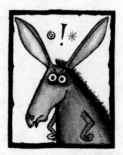

£30 would be nice. Thank you for trying! – *Michelle Varney, East Midlands*
Michelle, sweetie. It's a little more complicated than 'going out shopping with other people's money and having babies occasionally', darling. Perhaps when you outgrow your *penchant* for off-the-shoulder tops, you will understand. Until then, do your own donkey-work. Eeeeor ooooor.

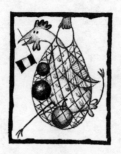

ablative
in latin the ablative is the
'kitchen drawer' of cases, where the
things that have no other natural home go
*a mélange of bits and bobs: where to find
cotton clerical shirts, Spanish fans, old-
fashioned school satchels,
skate gear, etc., etc., etc.*

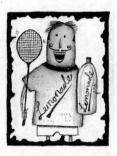

I am very environmentally aware and always try to buy clothes from companies that are 'green'. I do a lot of sports and remember reading of a company that did recycled polyester sports clothes. Do you know who I mean?
– T. Fox, Manchester

There are two companies I know of that do this: Patagonia and Karrimor. They both make fleecy tops and bottoms from recycled plastic bottles. When I first heard of this I imagined some sort of futuristic-looking garment woven out of shredded plastic, but they are nothing like this. There is no way you could tell; they just look like nice, soft, fleecy clothes and are very comfortable to wear and stylish to look at. (But make great conversation pieces – 'Guess what this is made of?') For stockist information and a catalogue for Patagonia, call 0033 141101818. For Karrimor, call 01254 893000. If you are interested in green things you may also like to know about Greenfibres, a mail-order company who do organic cotton clothes for men, women and children, and babies' nappies. Call 01803 868001 for a catalogue.

I wear leggings nearly all the time, but find that after only a short while they break around the inside leg seam. I'm only a size 12 so surely it can't be because I'm putting them under great strain?
– Paula Mitchell, Merseyside

No, of course not. Most leggings break because they're crap, have no seam allowance to speak of and no gusset. You need to look for a pair that has a diamond gusset (essential for movement so that the strain isn't taken by the seams; this has nothing to do with how big you are, but unless you intend standing still all day you will open and close your legs, even if just to walk) and is very well made, with fibres such as Supplex and/or Lycra for stretch and comfort. Marks & Spencer can't really be beaten in this. They always have some in: sizes 8–18, prices from about £15.

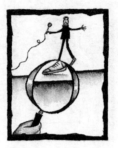

I recently went to see the Pet Shop Boys on their 'Somewhere' tour at the Savoy Theatre. During the interval, the Pet Shop Boys changed. They started off the second half wearing blue outfits and fantastic trainers. As I was sitting quite close to the back, I could not see the make of the trainers. I would be ever so grateful if you could find out the make and a possible stockist for me. – *Miss Mary Foster, East Sussex*

Well, I tried two avenues here. I contacted eminent author/ respected journalist and general world authority on the PSB, Chris Heath, for help. He never replied. Naughty Chris! But I let him off because I believe he was busy making soup for his girlfriend and travelling the world writing big articles. Then I contacted someone from their record label and they said, 'They're from that shop in Neal Street, I think it's called Buffalo.' And, indeed, there is a shop in Covent Garden called Buffalo that sells funky trainers. Their number is 0171 240 0605. So, Miss Mary, be ever so grateful, but you'll have to make a trip to London if you want to look like Neil or the other one from this fine British pop group.

Do you have any inside tips on what will be big for spring '99?
– *Helen Avanti, Cornwall*

Rock-climbing shoes, nurses' frilly-cuff things that you wear on your upper arm, pens worn with cord around the neck, clutch bags that look like rolled magazines, duffel coats, fishermen's waistcoats, Case Logic portable CD bags used as 'everyday' bags and brooches. I made all this up but just you wait and see.

I keep reading of knee boots, but where can one get boot trees to keep them looking good? I can't find them anywhere.
– *Kitty Hanning, Crystal Palace*

Johnny Loulou do some for £9.95; they are called the Dascomat boot shaper. Another place to look is antique shops, as they often have the most beautiful old-fashioned wooden ones. And you are right, boot trees and shoe trees should really be used to keep one's posher footwear in tip-toe condition.

Where can I get velvet jeans from? – *Emma Bennett, London*
The mail-order company Boden (0181 453 1535) do a lovely pair, in sizes 8–16, in various colours that change seasonally.

I like wearing T-shirts under casual shirts (with one button undone so you can see them), but mine always end up looking very saggy around the neck. Do you know of any good-quality ones that will last a bit longer? *–Michael Whatley, London*
I used to watch *CHIPs* on a Saturday and wish for an immaculately pressed and snug around the neck T-shirt like Eric Estrada wore. It looked so fine under his pale blue policeman's shirt. And I too used to end up with saggy-necked T-shirts. This is because I wore the wrong type (and also was loath to iron it, thus making it worse). There are two types of T-shirt I think (possibly more, but two will do for now): the sort you wear under a shirt, which should be snug, and the sort you wear on its own, which can also be snug, of course, but usually it is made in cotton and is baggier. The snug type is the sort you see men who work out in the gym wearing when they are not in the gym. I think you'd like a range called JCT by John Crummay, 43–45 Shorts Gardens, London WC2H 9AP, tel: 0171 240 3534; it is a basic T-shirt range and prices start at £49. He uses Diabolo, Tactel and Lycra fibres.

I own a lovely old silver-filigree belt buckle, which I enjoy wearing both in the daytime and in the evening. Unfortunately, the black suede leather belt to which it is attached is in need of replacing. Can you please advise me on where to have this done? – *Judith Beadle, Surrey*
Well, I spoke to a lovely lady at Frogpool Manor Saddlery on 0181 300 0716. They normally work in bulk for the equestrian world, but they could make you a belt in bridle-back leather from £18 and with suede stitched on to it from £24 (it depends obviously on length and width). It would take two to three weeks and colours are fairly limited (black and two types of brown).

As an arthritic octogenarian I must keep warm, but I am not comfortable in trousers. In winter I wear long johns and I need to replace them. Can you tell me if anyone in this area still stocks them? Or can you supply a mail-order address? I shall appreciate your help. – *Winifred Smith (Mrs), London*

Marks & Spencer do a truly brilliant thermal range called Active 2000 in sizes 8–20 in black or white, in long johns, short-sleeved T-shirts and long-sleeved ones. Really good, I thoroughly recommend them for total toastiness.

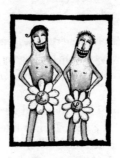

My partner and I are street flower-sellers in Manchester city centre. We provide a range of diverse and high-quality flowers. We have been saving for the past six months for new wardrobes. Our budget is limited to around £1,000, but we understand we can slowly extend our wardrobe over the years by specializing in a definite image. We shall be in London in early February and wish to know where we can buy quality second-hand 1930s–1950s suits, or second-hand designer clothes, unusual and exotic accessories, especially cravats, cufflinks, shirts and shoes. Alternatively, we know a good tailor in Manchester who with the right material will make suits to our specifications. Where are there drapers' shops with an exciting and unusual range of suit cloth?
– Gerard McDermott and Bennett Mott, Manchester

When I'm next in Manchester I shall call on you and pick up some flowers, which I hope you will give me a jolly big discount on. Shops to visit for all your requirements: Steinberg and Tolkein, 193 King's Road, sw3 (Sloane Square tube, near Chelsea Register Office), tel: 0171 376 3660; Cenci, 31 Monmouth Street, wc2 (Covent Garden tube), tel: 0171 836 1400, then try Blackout II, 51 Endell Street, wc2 (also Covent Garden tube), tel: 0171 240 5006; High Society, 46 Cross Street, n1 (Highbury and Islington or Angel tube), tel: 0171 226 6863; Crazy Clothes Connection, 134 Lancaster Road, w11 (Ladbroke Grove tube), tel: 0171 221 3989; then Merchant of Europe, 232 Portobello Road, w11 (Ladbroke Grove tube), tel: 0171 221 4203; and lastly, Bertie Wooster, 284 Fulham Road, sw6 (Earl's Court or Fulham Broadway tube), tel: 0171 352 5662. As for fabric shops, try Berwick Street, w1

(Oxford Circus tube), as they have a few good shops; Harrods
(Knightsbridge tube), Selfridges (Marble Arch or Bond Street tube)
and Liberty (Oxford Circus tube) – then go on to Berwick Street,
as it's just round the corner. [For more hints on fabric, have a look
in the 'Sew, Sew' chapter.]

My girlfriend has lovely long hair but cannot find a decent bathing cap to

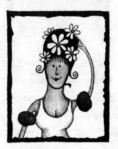

**wear in our municipal swimming pool. Unlike most women, she wants to
protect her hair from the chlorine in the water which gives her split ends
and ruins its fine nature. Most bathing caps are old-fashioned and make
her look like a pinhead! The ones on sale in the baths in machines (no not
THOSE machines) are thin and designed for women with perfect oval features – or mannequins. They don't really flatter her. She wants a cap that
will give her a bit of height on the top of her head. Colour/pattern are less
important. Bathing caps do not seem to have kept pace with other sportswear or swimwear. As you can see at any pool, most women put style
before haircare and simply do not wear a cap at all. Any ideas?**
– Richard Lysons, Bury

I cannot tell you how stylish *I* look in my Speedo silicon cap,
high-necked swimsuit and mirrored goggles, and I put performance before how I look any swimming day of the week. I can't
help thinking it's a bit naff to worry that much about how you
look when you swim. Most swimming caps make people look like
they have a pinhead – to get height, one must wear synchronized-
swimming-style hats with lots of frou-frou flowers (and isn't that
just another way of looking ridiculous?). For something a bit different, try some of these shops: Lilywhites, London w1, and
Mundy Sports, London n10; for vintage ones, try Delta of Venus
(0171 387 3037) and Greenwich Market. There is also a fabulously
cheeky catalogue of Björn Borg designs (0171 937 2226), among
which are some rather superb examples of swimmy headwear. My

hunch is that she'll find what she wants from vintage shops – she'll have to hunt around though.

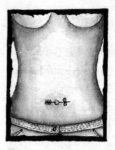

Pierced noses, navels, eyebrows and increasingly lips and cheeks are commonplace these days. I had my navel pierced a few years ago and have taken up my previously failed search of finding something other than rings or bars for my pierced belly-button. I'm sure lots of people with pierced body parts would be keen to have new and different pieces in the same way that we all like to change our earrings, rings and necklaces. The distinct lack of choice also applies to practical body jewellery. Everyone with a pierced navel has suffered bouts of inflammation and I believe this is due to clothing catching on jewellery which is bulky and can easily cause infection. Do you know of anywhere that specializes in body jewellery, or somewhere that will design and make jewellery out of surgical steel for my purposes? – *Jeannette Crockett, London N7*

The Wildcat Body Collection do all sorts of ready-made nice stuff and they do a catalogue, so write to 16 Preston Street, Brighton, East Sussex BN1 2HN, or telephone on 01273 323758, saying for what part of the body you need jewellery. Their products are made of surgical steel, 18ct gold or niobium, which is a hypo-allergenic material that comes in different colours and does not affect the skin. Jess James, 3 Newburgh Street, London W1V 1LH, tel: 0171 437 0199, will make things up for you wherever technically possible, in silver, 18ct gold or platinum, but not surgical steel. Prices start at £100. Finally, Into You, 144 St John Street, London EC1V 4UA, tel: 0171 253 5085, can also make things up to your own design in 18ct gold or white gold; prices start at £60. Nobody I spoke to recommended surgical steel for your own designs, but I hope that the places I've mentioned will open up more choice for you.

I am having a few problems finding American-type 'skate gear' and was hoping you could help. I am a sixteen-year-old girl and a size 6–8. I live in Preston but will travel to Manchester or near by. I will also be visiting London some time soon. I would be so grateful if you could inform me of stockists in these areas as I desperately need some new clothes for summer. Pleeease help! – *Suzanne Marsden, Bamber Bridge, Preston*

Exit (Unit 1, Affleck's Arcade, Manchester, tel: 0161 832 4028) stocks 'hardcore' skate labels, straight from America, including East Coast and DC. They stock X-Girl, which is exclusively for girls (T-shirts cost around £19.95), and Kanabeach, Soochi, Hooch Fehm, Cyberdog and E Pure. The small size would be right for you. In London the place to go is Slam City Skates (16 Neal's Yard, WC2, tel: 0171 240 0928, Covent Garden tube), which stocks Stussy, Volcon, Holmes and Fresh Jive for girls. If you can't get there in person, they do a mail-order service if you know exactly what you want, and you'll also need your ma or pa's credit card (yeah!!); p&p varies depending on what is being sent (*c.* £3 for a T-shirt). Before I get complaining letters, I am aware that these are big prices for a teenager, but skate gear is expensive. OK?

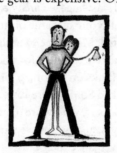

Why is it that one can't buy any decent dresses with pockets nowadays? For several weekends recently my wife has taken me shopping to help her choose a nice new summer dress, but every time we found something with a decent fabric and style that looked promising, she rejected it because it had no pockets. A few years ago it seemed that two-thirds of dresses had pockets, but now it is about 0.1 per cent. Why is this? Are women expected to carry a handbag if all they need is a hanky? My wife is thirty-nine and a fairly standard size 10/12; she likes cotton dresses with lots of flare, in below-the-knee lengths. This should not be a difficult requirement! Can you suggest any good stores to try? I would never think of buying trousers without pockets, so why are women expected to accept dresses without them? – *Gareth G. Morgan, York*

Oh, goodness, Gareth, who knows? I guess dresses are taking part
in that thing called evolution too. You know, few women take han-
kies with them now, so the dresses think, 'Why bother?' I am very
partial to a real hanky, and I always make my husband carry mine.
If for no other reason than that I can stick my hand down his front
pocket when I get a runny nose (which I do often, 'specially when
eating soup). Nightingales (call 0870 601 2415 for mail order) have
lots of pretty dresses that I think your wife will like and many of
the models are standing with their hands in their pockets, so the
dresses must have them. All very reasonably priced. Racing Green
(0990 411 1111) also always have lovely dresses that definitely have
side pockets. So, how will you spend your weekends now?

**This request is so pathetically ordinary that only desperation makes me
expose myself to ridicule by sending it. Where can I buy well-made, elegant
silk, cotton or linen shirts in bright jewel or pastel colours? Not browns, not
oranges, not sludges of any hue, not big overshirts – just tailored shirts to
wear with suits? I have shopped in Knightsbridge, Bond Street, Oxford
Street – not to mention the Boulevard Saint-Germaine and the entire 6th
arrondissement. You are my last hope. – *Christine, via e-mail***
Well, Christine, I have left your surname off to save you ridicule,
although none is warranted. Madeleine Hamilton makes 'quality tailored shirts for women' that are perfect for under suits. Most need
cufflinks, but I think cufflinks on a woman look divine. (Or man for
that matter. When I worked Somewhere Else, I had the most massive
crush on a man named Robert, who wore divine blue shirts, ironed to
within an inch of their lives, and he always wore cufflinks. He was
much older than I, and ever since then I can barely look at a cufflink
without remembering his deep commanding voice saying, 'Have you
finished?' as we met by the photocopier . . . sigh.) Well, this
Madeleine woman can make shirts to order but says there is usually
no need as they are sized XS–L (or 8–16), and they can be altered. No
bright jewel colours but plenty of pastels, including five shades of
baby blue, lilac and pink. Mail order available, although selection is
more limited (call on 0171 404 8484 for more info). Thomas Pink do
a label called 'Ladies' fitted' in four colours, including light green and
white, which are available mail order, tel: 0171 498 3882, and have
stores in Jermyn Street, London SW1Y 6JD, and others in London,
Dublin, Edinburgh and Glasgow. If you want my advice, though,
Chrissie, and you obviously do, get the bugger made for you.

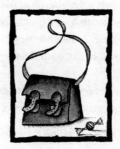

I am desperate for an old-fashioned school leather satchel. I want the kind with a shoulder strap and two pockets at the front. It must be big enough to hold an A4 folder (preferably two). Please can you help me, as I have absolutely no idea where to buy one. If you could I would be eternally grateful! – *Rachel Tomlinson, Cowbridge, South Wales*

Aren't they lovely, those old leather satchels? Some flash bag designers do posh versions of them that can run into thousands, but if you want a good old-fashioned one, then go to any of Johnny Loulou's stores (such as Peter Jones). In their luggage department (and sometimes in schoolwear) they do leather satchels with two front pockets. I don't know if it would be big enough to take your files, but I guess you could always pop down with your files and do a bit of surreptitious stuffing. They cost £35. Eden's, a specialist schoolwear shop in Talbot Green (01443 223387), were nice and helpful. They said that they can get what you want from a leather-goods maker who supplies their two shops; prices start at £59.99, but they reckon they can get exactly the right thing, so it's worth giving them a call.

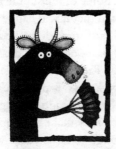

Since a recentish trip to Spain, I have become thoroughly converted to the wisdom of carrying a fan with me at all times, especially in the summer, especially on the tube. However, I have just lost my last Spanish fan and don't know where to start looking for them in the UK. Can you suggest

anywhere, preferably in London, Edinburgh or Glasgow, that sells reason-
able-quality contemporary Spanish fans (not frilly tourist souvenirs and
definitely not Far Eastern paper or balsa fans, which just don't do the job
at all)? I'd be happy to pay up to £15 each. Thank you very much.
– *Jane Adams, Edinburgh*

Catherine Darcy (01273 477699) imports them for use on stage and
has a stack of antique and modern ones, for £10 + p&p.

Clergy do not have a great range of attire. It has improved since the Church
of England started ordaining women to the priesthood, but there is still a
long way to go. Particularly difficult are shirts. Most clergy shirts are made
of poly-cotton, which, not to put too fine a point on it, tend to smell
appallingly in the summer, when they come into contact with perspiration.
Clerical shirts also tend to be rather old-fashioned in the way they are cut.
Until my ordination I had worn M&S 100 per cent cotton shirts for years and
I loved them. What I long for is a good-quality 100 per cent cotton clerical
shirt with a tonsure collar, button cuffs and a breast pocket that has a little
row of stitches that makes a pen compartment. Is there any hope? Or do I
pray that clerical shirts become a fashion item next season and M&S will
start making them so that I can buy in a lifetime's supply? Any help in finding the ideal clerical shirt would be most appreciated.
– *Reverend Richard Curtis, Leicester*

The reason that clerical shirts are now increasingly made in poly-
cotton is because they are easier to care for and – so I'm told by
people who know these things – men aren't very good at looking
after their shirts. Sexist? I know. Not to mention the fact that there
are women priests now. But wait! Apparently there is a swing back
to wanting cotton shirts. Some of the suppliers I spoke to are
working on it, so pray hard that it will happen. But wait some
more! Wippell's (clerical outfitters) do make a pure-cotton, tonsure-collar shirt with a breast pocket and dual cuffs! The Lord has
heard our prayers already, Richard. Available in black only, for
£44, ref. no. 945 (call 0171 222 4528 and state collar size; be ready
with a deposit, because they are made to order). There is another
supplier in Rome – maybe they make the Pope's shirts, ooooh! –
but you shouldn't need to go so far afield now. Pronto! Pronto!

And here are some more:

In answer to the plea of the Reverend Richard Curtis, here are two suppliers
of pure-cotton clerical shirts. L. J. Shirts of Unit 07c, Oakwood House, 422

Hackney Road, London E2 7SY, tel: 0171 729 4124, did me some tonsure-collar pure-cotton shirts for just under £25 which were very serviceable. For the luxury feel of superfine cotton, Seymours' shirts from 136 Sunbridge Road, Bradford BD1 2QG, tel: 01274 726520, do some at £55 (for all you fellow clergy, I bought two with my ordination grant a few years ago). – *Cheryl Collins, Sheffield*

Thank you so much, Cheryl. I'm sure Richard (if I may be so informal) will find this most helpful.

This is not strictly a fashion problem but I would be grateful if you can offer any help. I am trying to find a hanging clothes bag in which dresses or suits can be transported on their hangers and will take half a dozen or so garments. Any ideas about where I might look? My sons use them for taking clothes to and from university digs, and it saves folding and packing into suitcases. Your column is full of useful and fascinating tips – one of the first things I turn to in the paper! – *Mrs J. Campbell, London*

I know what you mean. Johnny Loulou do smaller hanging bags, as do lots of other places, but not one that holds lots. Morplan are suppliers to the trade of all things to do with retail and ordinary mortals can also go in and buy from their shop at 56 Great Titchfield Street, London W1P 8DX. Enquiries: 0800 435333. They have a few suitables. If you want something that really lasts, then go for their Garment Carrying Bag, which is excellent. I used to use one when I was a lowly fashion assistant and it held lots (about twenty-five garments, so maybe a bit much for you) and put up with lots of tantrumy behaviour: in three sizes, from £145 exclusive of VAT (expensive, I know, but it's more like a travelling wardrobe; you can even padlock it). Or try their Sample Garment Bag, made from blue nylon. There are several lengths, holding ten to twenty garments; prices from £5.39 each, again exclusive. Or they do the Repsac, which holds up to twenty-five garments and starts at £31.50, exclusive.

I do hope you can help me. A little while ago, having just given birth to my second baby, I was feeling a little low and postnatal (as you do). A rather perky little size 8 friend of mine popped round to cheer me up. This she failed to do, being so perky and gorgeous, but I coveted a rather cunning bag she had just bought, and have been searching for said bag ever since. It is just Filofax size, with a zip all the way around, and in it are various compartments for mobile phone, keys, etc. – all the stuff that I don't haul around in my v. unfashionable baby-changing bag, but none the less I

would love to own such a gal-about-town item. She says it costs about £16 and came from somewhere in the West End. Can you help?
– *Abby Hoffmann, via e-mail, London*

I do believe it is the Wonderbag, £16 from branches of Debenhams and House of Fraser branches.

gold stars
awarded for the very best

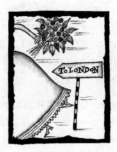

Gold Stars are the fashion equivalent of the Michelin stars. They go to people, shops and labels that I have personal experience of for being excellent; the entries explain in more detail exactly why. This chapter uses very varied problems to introduce the Gold Star holder and it is not arranged in any particular order. Gold Star holders are all equally brilliant and no higher accolade can be granted.

I'd like to buy my girlfriend an engagement ring, but haven't a huge amount of money. I don't want to buy her one of those tiny diamonds but thought you could recommend something unusual to make up for my lack of money! – *Tom de Victor, London*

Oh, you sweet man for not just going and buying some apple-pip diamond from Argos and giving it to her over a Harvester dinner. Sure, it's nice to have a stonking diamond on your finger, but it's also nice to have enough money to pay the rent and buy tea-bags. **The Gold Star award here goes to Jess James**, 3 Newburgh Street, London WIL ILH , tel: 0171 437 0199. Not only do they stock lots of jewellery designers, but they also have their own designs and will work to commission. Jess Canty, who owns Jess James, revolutionized the jewellery industry when he opened his shop ten years ago with his fresh approach. None of that stuffy, scary business you normally associate with 'proper' jewellers. Although he trades in a lot of modern silver designs, you can also get gold, antiquey things. His ideas and designs are innovative and classy and his shop is absolutely worth a visit. It is cram-packed with great ideas, from the very reasonably priced to the more expensive. Jess does something called prayer rings, which are destined to become new classics because they are masterpieces of engineering – nuggets of white gold, yellow gold and platinum which you fiddle with and swivel round. It's not perhaps right for an engagement present but it

would make a great alternative to a wedding band. They cost
£1,200 and are worth every penny. There is also a chunky catalogue
full of photos if you want to buy by mail order, but for (especially)
anyone planning to get married a trip to London to Jess James is
highly recommended.

**I need help with shoes. The real problem is in summer, as my feet are
sweaty. It's not my fault – it's genetic – we are a family of foot-sweaters. In
winter my socks and insoles look after the problem, but I really, really want
to be able to wear lightweight summer shoes without socks or tights. I tend
to wear either plimsole-type canvas shoes with insoles and keep washing
both, or strappy sandals which give enough draughts, plus insoles if not
too hideous, though nice sandals tend not to fit my fat feet. How can I wear
standard enclosed summer shoes? Has science come up with a solution?
Do foot deodorants work? The ones I tried years ago didn't make any difference. Are my summer outfits destined to look elegant to the ankles and
ridiculous thereafter for ever? Help me! – Jo Griggs, East Sussex**
I have no idea if foot deodorants work as, she says smugly, I have
never had any need for them. In fact, my feet have always been so
remarkably unsmelly that it has caused astonishment among my
friends. Once when I was on holiday with five girlfriends we all
bought the same flat canvas shoes. Towards the end of the holiday
all theirs stunk like an incontinent tramp's pants, but not mine. Of
course, you know about the merits of wearing footwear with
leather insoles rather than yukky perspiration-inducing synthetic
(quite a lot of the time shoes will have leather uppers and synthy
stuff next to your feet, which I think is quite, quite stupid). There
isn't a solution as such, just some suggestions. There will be times
when you have to wear enclosed shoes in the summer; for these
times I suggest you try the following: to stop the sweating, try a
product called Trust, which comes in a cream form in a very small
pot which lasts for ages and is, I have it on good authority, very
effective. You put it on about twice a week – putting it on
overnight and washing it off the next morning. After that you can
wash as many times as you like without affecting it until the next
'application'. It doesn't stop you sweating but ensures that your
sweat never smells. You can get it from places like Boots for about
£8. Or, if you decide you don't want to put stuff on your feet, try
wearing **Secret Socks, which are awarded the second Gold Star**,
because they are excellent. They will go some way to absorbing the

sweat and protect the shoes and you also won't need to wash your trainers and stuff so often. You know those hideous footlets you get that are the colour of old ladies' knickers? Well, Secret Socks are not like that because they are in thin towelling and are very 'discreet'. They come in black, white or beige, in sizes small (shoe sizes 1–4), medium (4–7), large (7–9) and extra large (10–13), and cost £1.99 per pair (mail order and enquiries: 0171 794 2066). I wear mine in the summer with my desert boots, in my trainers when I go to the gym and as an extra layer in winter. They wash up brilliantly and everyone should have some. Finally, try Sundaes (01406 371370). They make sandals to order [see their entry in the 'Big Shoe' directory at the back of the book], so even if your feet are 'fat', these will fit! Finally, when you take your shoes off and they are resting – even sandals – dust them with a bit of talc to absorb moisture and keep them fresh.

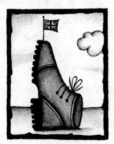

Since I retired I have developed a taste for more energetic holidays than the fortnight-flaked-out-on-a-beach that I needed as a working woman. My latest plan is a trip to Peru. The holiday notes advise a 'strong pair of walking boots'. I have never worn such a thing and the ones I have seen in the shops are almost too heavy to lift off the shelves, let alone attempt to lift up and down on the end of my feet. Could you find out for me please whether there are such things as strong but lightweight walking boots, and if so who sells them? My feet and I will be eternally grateful.
– *Maggie Paul, Esher, Surrey*

I love, love, love my **Ecco boots** ('Ecco boots, far away . . . da da . . . Ecco boots far away . . . da da . . .'). Hello. Yes, they are fantastic and **holders of Gold Star numero three.** I bought mine in Street in Somerset two years ago and they are light and wonderful but also tough and high-performing, with things like Gore-Tex linings (keep your feet from getting too hot – I even wear my boots in high summer with no discomfort – yet also keep them warm in winter). I'm not even going to bother recommending anyone else, because I know just what you mean about walking boots that are so heavy you never want to put them on. Here are a couple of styles you may like: Polden, which come in black/black and bison/black nubuck and costs £110, and Mendip, which come in coffee/black and bison/bison nubuck, also £110. Your nearest shop is the Ecco Shop, 18 White Lion Walk, Guildford, Surrey GU1 3DN, tel: 01483 302574. The stockist helpline number is 0800 387368. They may sound expensive but walking boots (proper ones) are. (Ecco boots actually inspired me to introduce the Gold Star system.)

I have turned to you in desperation! My beloved digital watch has finally given out after fourteen years and I can't find another one anywhere. I'm not particularly feminine but I don't want a monstrosity of a sports one like in the shops as I have a very small wrist and hand. I also would prefer a leather strap but I could change that. The absolute biggest size I could stand is about 2cm by 2cm and, please, something tasteful! My last watch was a Timex with a light and an alarm and something with those would be brilliant. Otherwise, up to £50 and anywhere in the country as I have relatives everywhere! – *Miriam Osner, Sheffield*

I find it hard to recommend anything, as digital watches should, to my mind, be worn big and chunky. Trying to mix digital displays with small, feminine styling looks yuk to me. I'd much rather you got yourself to Cobra and Bellamy (149 Sloane Street, London SW1X 9BZ, tel: 0171 730 9993) and bought yourself a lovely 'old-fashioned' watch with hands. They do a cheapie range (but frigging gorgeous) that starts at about the £39 mark. And here is where I launch into a story. About five years ago I went into Cobra and Bellamy in the course of my job, and found the watch I had been looking for all my life. It was silver with a long rectangular face, very Art Deco. I was obsessed with it but it cost around £600. Every time I spoke to Veronica (one of the owners) after that, I asked about this masterpiece of timekeeping. Then, about two years after I had first seen it, Veronica rang me one day at work and said, 'Guess what? That watch you like, we now make it in chrome plate rather than silver and the face is curved plastic [previously the face had been in glass and curved glass is very difficult and expensive to produce] and it's £59.' I almost flew down there. And it is just fabulous: it keeps time like a shop steward, is utterly beautiful and unique, and much remarked upon. I adore it. But this is just one watch in a fabulous range of beautiful watches for men and women that are beautifully styled and ridiculously well priced; for which **Cobra and Bellamy win a Gold Star.**

I am planning a holiday later this year and want to be able to swim. But I have an added problem when choosing a swimsuit as I had a mastectomy last year. I have heard that there are some companies that specialize in this area but feel apprehensive and don't know where to start looking.
– H. Everidge, Kingston

Please don't be apprehensive. Going on holiday and swimming are both positive steps after a mastectomy and your attitude is to be applauded. Naturally you don't know where to start looking because, thankfully, this isn't an area of swimsuits that you've ever had to worry about before. Mastectomy swimsuits have to be cleverly thought out as they can't be too low and have to be high-cut under the arms to conceal scarring. [Have a good look through the 'Swimwear' directory at the back of this book for a full selection of who does mastectomy swimwear (Fantasie, Splash Out and Rigby and Peller are three to look out for especially, but there are others).] Someone I'm going to recommend you see, above all others, is the excellent, the divine, the fabulous **Margaret Ann (01985 840520), holder of Gold Star number five.** Margaret Ann is an underwear/swimwear expert [for the full low-down, look at 'Swimwear' and 'Underwear' directories – she is in both]. She works with lots of post-mastectomy women and her service is superb; she has literally changed the lives of thousands of women. She doesn't just deal with mastectomy but with larger-than-average-sized swimwear, underwear, first bras – you name it, she does it. If a bra can be got in the world, she can get it. Margaret Ann is so excellent I think she should be knighted.

My husband and I are going on a long (three-month) trip across the States and maybe further afield. It will be fairly 'adventurous' in the sense that we'll be walking lots and maybe even do some rock-climbing! We'd like to get some 'outdoor' gear like fleeces, waterproofs, etc. and need your guidance as to what makes are really good. We won't be buying loads (this isn't a trip up Everest after all) but I do want them to be good quality. I have dreadful memories of buying an inferior ski jacket one winter and freezing to death. We're only in our thirties and I HATE patterns. Hope this isn't being too fussy. – Mr and Mrs Davies, Cornwall

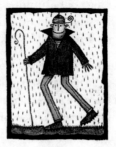

Good grief, you are not being fussy in the slightest. I *insist* on the highest-performance outdoor wear. I could have cried with frustration when fleeces (which naturally I had been wearing for ages) became . . . oh my goodness, I can barely say it . . . *fashionable.* And in the trail of this trendiness there were *fashion fleeces.* Look no further, my good woman, than my favourite, favourite label of all time: **Patagonia, Gold Star awardee number six.** I have oft joked to Mr Annie that I want to be buried wearing one of my Patagonia fleeces, but actually I rather fancy something a little smarter would be more apt. But enough of this talk. Patagonia was started in 1973 by people who fished/climbed rocks – that type of thing. Hence their stuff is not the cheapest, but it is superb. I can spot a piece of Patagonia clothing from fifty paces and it quickens my heartbeat every time. I have about ten of their fleeces, in various weights and for various conditions, and all are excellent. For your trip I'd particularly recommend the Retro Cardigan (a fabulous, slightly fitted fleece with zip front) and the Retro-X waistcoat, which is wind-proof. I also have their silk-weight long johns and zip turtle neck, their neck gaiters, their bags, their Bunting gloves, all their fishing stuff . . . etc., etc. This is a cliché, but I cannot recommend Patagonia enough – they are a class apart. Call 0033 141101818 for their catalogue (you can do mail order or ring that number for your nearest stockist, but I'd go the mail-order route; you'll have a far better choice) and get drooling.

**the
directories**

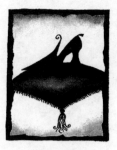

big shoe

'Big Shoe' has become a bit of a misnomer since this directory now covers all sorts. From orthopaedic needs to narrow, wide, bridal, made to measure and vegan. But for old times' sake I wanted to keep it as the 'Big Shoe' directory. These shops are listed either because they responded to a cry for help – to make themselves known – or because readers recommended them. Some of those listed work from showrooms or workshops (i.e., not all those listed are retail shops as such), so I advise ringing first to make an appointment. **Nationwide** covers brands that are stocked throughout the country; ring for your nearest stockists or dedicated mail order. But lots of those listed also do mail order, so it's worth having a good read through all the entries.

NATIONWIDE

Joseph Cheaney and Sons Ltd
Rushton Road, Desborough, Kettering,
Northants NN14 2RZ
T 01536 760383
J. Cheaney makes men's Goodyear
welted footwear in sizes 6–12 (all styles)
and sizes 6–15 (some styles). There are
stockists all over the UK, and mail
orders can be delivered within a week.
Prices are at the top end of the market.

Start-Rite Shoes
T 0800 783 2138 for stockist/catalogue
enquiries and advice line
Premium shoes for children in six width
fittings. Sizes start at infant size 2 right
up to adult size 10, in widths D–H;
though not every size in every width,
most sizes are stocked in three width fittings. Prices start at £12 (canvas shoes)
and £25 (first shoes). The Inneraze range
gives extra support for children with
walking difficulties such as pronation.
Doctor's referral is recommended.
Prices from £32.

Sundaes
The Chase, 18 High Street, Moulton,
Spalding, Lincs PE12 6QB
T 01406 371370
Sundaes is a mail-order company which
makes sandals and can also supply
Haflinger wool felt slippers and clogs
for ladies, men and children. Ladies' are
sized 3–10, men's 6–12. Prices
£31.95–£49.95. There is a colour
catalogue and the mail-order service is
international.

EAST ANGLIA

Carter's Shoes
2 Comberton Road, Barton,
Cambridge CB3 7BA
T 01223 264930
Carter's specialize in very narrow- and
very wide-fitting shoes for men and
women. Ladies' shoe sizes from 2–10
(AA–EEE) and are priced between £45
and £90. Men's from 5–13 (E–G) and
cost £40–£120. The shop is near to
Junction 12 of the M11 (South East
area); stock changes constantly so they
advise ringing first to discuss specific
requirements.

Momo the Cobbler
8 Cobble Yard, Napier Street,
Cambridge CB1 1HR
T 01223 358209
Momo makes all types of shoes (walk-
ing/sandals/formal) for all types of people (men/women/children/orthopaedic)
in all sizes. This comprehensive range
starts at £120. No mail order.

LONDON

Amanda Norris
Studio based in Islington
T 0181 986 0087 for enquiries
Bespoke shoes for men, women and
children. Children's sizes 5–12, adult
sizes 2–12/13. From initial consultation
to discuss shape, leather, etc., it takes
four to five weeks. Prices from £180 for
first pair with £50 deposit. Appointments necessary.

Anello & Davide
47 Beauchamp Place, London SW3 1NX
T 0171 225 2468; call for details of
nationwide stockists too
Bridal, evening and designer shoes for
women in sizes 3–8. Shoes can also be
made to order (prices start at £150–£225
for bridal but can vary widely according
to materials used; and £175 upwards for
other types of shoe) in colour or material
of client's choice. A mail-order service
and catalogue are available.

Baboucha Shoes and Bags
218 High Street, Barnet, Herts EN5 5SZ
T 0181 441 3788
Third-generation shoemakers at
Baboucha produce any type of shoes
(orthopaedic, elevated, historical,
theatrical, fetish and vegan to name
but a few), for any type of feet (men's,
women's, oddly sized) in any size. They
also dye fabric and leather shoes. There
is no mail order or catalogue. Home
consultations are chargeable and it takes
six to eight weeks for made-to-measure
shoes. Prices start at £250.

Birkenstock Shop
37 Neal Street, London WC2H 9PR
T 0171 240 2783
Birkenstock offer 'foot-shaped' sandals
and shoes in leather, suede and a vegan
alternative, Birkoflor. Birkis start at
£29.95, the vegan selection starts at
£42.95. Sizes 24–46. Insoles available.
mail-order catalogue available (0800
132194).

Connolly
32 Grosvenor Crescent Mews,
London SW1X 7EX
T 0171 235 3883
Very high-quality moccasins, loafers, driving shoes and boots (with crêpe soles)
for men and women. Connolly make the
original Car Shoe – designed in the 1960s
– with its distinctive rubber studs on the
underside; it is made from a single piece
of leather and is hand-stitched. Sizes
range from 35–46, prices £195–£250.
Catalogue available for mail order.

Deliss
15 St Alban's Grove, London W8 5BP
T 0171 938 2255
Deliss make made to measure all types
of shoes for all types of feet (including
orthopaedic). All sizes can be made.
Prices start at £390 for ladies' shoes and
£470 for men's.

G. J. Cleverley
12 Royal Arcade, Old Bond Street,
London W1X 3HB
T 0171 493 0443/1058
Bespoke shoes made in any leather,
predominantly men's. Customer is
asked exactly what he wants, it takes
three to six months, any size catered
for. Prices from £1,000. Will travel to
visit their customers.

Hanna Goldman Shoes
Studio 4, 10–13 Hollybush Place,
London E2 9QX
T 0171 739 2690
Ladies' wedding shoes, evening shoes,
shoes for any special occasion are made
to order. Sizes 1–12. Prices start at £195.
They have a brochure costing £3.

Helen Creedy Smith Shoes
c/o Edwina Ibbotson Millinery,
45 Queenstown Road, London SW8 3RG
T 0171 498 5390
Very unusual bridal shoes for the more
modern bride and special-occasion shoes,
for women. Sizes 3–8 1/2. Prices start at
£225 for shoes and £350 for boots.

James Taylor and Son
4 Paddington Street, London W1M 3LA
T 0171 935 4149 for enquiries/brochure
Handmade men's and ladies' shoes to
measure in any size for large or problem
feet. Prices from £795 + VAT (first pair),
thereafter £595 from personal last. It
takes three months with fittings before
the shoes are complete; subsequent pairs
can be sent out by mail. In addition to a
'Rogues' Gallery' of odd shoes, there are
also some ready-to-wear shoes in stock
in sizes up to 13/14. Shoes can be adapted
and customized: e.g. arch supports
added, shoes stretched, etc.

Leatherworks
77–79 Southgate Road, London N1 3HZ
T 0171 359 9778
Stilettos and platform shoes can be made to requirements. Can cater for the theatre and transvestites. Stilettos available in sizes 3–12 from £65. Lasts can be bought from £300 and are available up to size 14. Catalogues available from the above number, price £3.

Magnus of Northampton
63 Southend Road, London NW3 2QB
T 0171 435 1792
44 Chiltern Street, London W1M 1HG
T 0171 224 3938
Magnus have manufacturers worldwide who make shoes to their orders. They supply men's and women's formal and casual shoes and slippers. Men's are sized 12 to 16 and women's are sized 9 to 11. Prices to suit all pockets. There is a mail-order service and a free catalogue (one for men and one for women, state which one you want). There is also a shop in Northampton [see Midlands section].

The Natural Shoe Store
325 King's Road, London SW3 5ES
T 0171 351 3721
21 Neal Street, London WC2H 9PU
T 0171 836 5254
The Natural Shoe Store offers a variety of brands. Simple designs, practical construction and high-quality materials. Children's booties from £14.95, adults from £29.95. Sizes 35–46. Mail order available (0800 132194).

The Orthopaedic Footwear Co. Ltd at James Taylor and Son Bespoke Shoemakers
4 Paddington Street, London W1M 3LA
T 0171 935 4149
Every type of shoe is made here, including walking boots, sandals, formal shoes, golf shoes and riding boots – everyone is catered for. The size range is almost 0–60. Factory-made shoes start at £250, handmade start at £795 + VAT. There is a catalogue and although there is no mail order, they can post the shoes home

after the first visit; home visits are sometimes carried out. They also make foot supports and can customize people's own shoes.

Rochester Big and Tall
90 Brompton Road, London SW3 1ER
T 0171 838 0018
Rochester sells a wide range of shoes for men only. In sizes 10–16, width fittings D to WWW. Freephone for a catalogue (0800 442277).

The Small and Tall Shoe Shop
71 York Street, London W1H 2BJ
T 0171 723 5321
A full range of women's footwear in sizes 8 1/2 to 12 in width fittings AA to D. And small sizes 12 1/2 to 3 1/2. Prices £60–£85.

Special Feetures
Lion House, 27 High Street,
Thames Ditton, Surrey KT7 0SD
T 0181 398 8810
Mail-order company supplying long and narrow-fitting shoes for women only, everything from 'courts to sports'. Sizes go up to UK 11 1/2 in widths AAAA–B. The mail order covers the UK and the EU, but there is also a small showroom where customers can have their size checked (by appointment only), see the whole range and buy shoes. Call for a free brochure, which also includes a size-fitting chart. Prices £39–£79 approx.

Tony's of Fulham
7 Salisbury Pavement, Dawes Road,
London SW6 7HT
T 0171 381 4513
Hand-sewn traditional shoes, boots, riding boots and sandals to any size and width. Men's, women's and orthopaedic shoes. Hand-sewn traditional shoes start from £650; semi-traditional start from £350; ordinary machine-sewn from £275 and ladies' shoes from £210.

Trickers Shoemakers
67 Jermyn Street, London SW1Y 6NY
T 0171 930 6395
Trickers have a large selection of leathers

and styles from which men's made-to-measure shoes can be made. Walking boots and more formal styles can be made from approx. £185. Slippers and shoes also available from stock. Sizes 5–13+ can be made to special order. A mail-order catalogue is available.

MIDLANDS

Church and Company Footwear Ltd
Church's Shoes
St James, Northampton NN5 5JB
T 01604 751251
Church's make traditional men's shoes, including brogues, Oxfords, monks, Derbys, etc. Sizes range from 5 to 13 with a range of different width fittings. There is a catalogue and a mail-order service available (01323 730532 for details) which covers the whole of the UK and the world. Prices start at £200.

Grenson Shoes Ltd
Upper Queen Street, Rushden, Northants NN10 0AB
T 01933 358734
Grenson make formal, welted and bespoke shoes and boots for men and women. Women's shoes come in sizes 3–9, men's in 5–15. There is a catalogue available and customers can ring for details of nationwide stockists.

Harry Parkes Ltd
159 Corporation Street, Birmingham B4 6PH
T 0121 236 5476
As well as retailing regular-sized women's and children's shoes, Harry Parkes sell men's large sizes, up to size 16 or 17 in some lines. They are a sports shop, so they stock trainers and football, rugby and cricket boots. Mail order is available, although there is no catalogue. Prices £30–£120.

Magnus of Northampton
2 High Street, Harpole, Northampton NN7 4DH
T 01604 831271
Open 10 a.m.–4 p.m., Mon–Fri.
See entry in 'London' section.

SCOTLAND

Lewis Stuart
2 Rosemount Place, Aberdeen AB25 2XW
T 01224 630663
Lewis Stuart make orthopaedic walking shoes to any size. They also make basic shoes for ladies (i.e., not court shoes) and gents. Prices £300+. There is a catalogue and mail order is provided.

James Inglis
Eastwalk House, Eastgate, Peebles, Peebleshire EH45 8AD
T 01721 720781
James Inglis is predominantly a mail-order company selling narrow-fitting shoes, although you can buy all types of fittings at the shop at the above address. The size range is from 3–10 with half-sizes also available. Prices are wide-ranging: £39–£270. Mail-order catalogues come out twice a year and include several makes which are exclusive to them.

SOUTH EAST

The Glass Slipper
7 The High Street, Tunbridge Wells, Kent TN1 1UL
T 01892 511464
All types of shoes for women. Sizes 1–12 in B and C width fittings. A catalogue and mail-order service are available. Prices £50–£110.

SOUTH WEST

Bill Bird
49 Northwick Business Centre, Blockley, Glos GL56 9RF
T 01386 700855
Specialize in classic made-to-measure neat and elegant leather shoes that are also light and comfy to wear. Mr Bird studied chiropody better to understand foot disorders. He can make any style or size of shoe to order for all types of foot problems, large or small. Prices £395–£500 for shoes, plus £210 for your individual hand-carved last.

The Celtic Sheepskin Co.
**Wesley Yard, Newquay,
Cornwall TR7 1LB
T 01637 871605**
They make shoes for everyone and specialize in sheepskin boots, slippers and
leather sandals. They come in twenty-
four colours and any special requirements can be catered for. Sizes from a
child's 5 to adult 14. Prices £15–£65. A
worldwide mail-order service is available,
with a catalogue.

Charles Macwatt Originals:
Handmade Boots and Shoes
**7 Christmas Steps, Bristol, BS1 5BS
T 0117 9214247**
Emphasis is placed on providing a perfect
fit for customers with specific foot difficulties, as well as offering a large selection
of leathers and designs. Small, large, narrow, wide, orthopaedic, odd-sized feet,
made to measure – all are covered. Shoes
are handmade in the workshop so there is
maximum flexibility. Standard adult
sizes, 2–14 (AA width for sizes 2–11 1/2
and E–H for sizes 2–14). Children's from
small 4 to youth's 5 1/2 in C–H fittings.
Prices from £34. Telephone for a free catalogue.

Conker Shoe Company
**83 High Street, Totnes, Devon TQ9 5PB
T 01803 862490**
Conker Shoe make all types of footwear
(shoes, sandals, boots, casual, bespoke),
and they cater for men, women, children
and those with orthopaedic problems.
Shoes are made to suit individual
requirements following standard designs.
Sizes start at 7 (children's) through to
adult 13 (half-sizes available) in four
widths. Prices £33–£90 for standard
sizes. They are based in the South West
but cover all the UK and abroad via mail
order – a free catalogue is available.

Crispian Shoemakers
**Bell Hill, Norton St Philip, Bath BA3 6LT
T 01373 834639**
They sell comfortable, foot-shaped shoes
for women and men with 'normal' or

problem feet. It is a family business and
all shoes can be made to measure in their
small workshop. They specialize in well-
made sandals, boots and shoes using the
finest materials. Prices £50–£300.

Event
**17 New Bond Street, Bath BA1 1BA
T 01225 481103**
Event stock men's and women's shoes in
fashionable styles. Sizes 37–42 in
women's and 41–46 in men's, prices
£35–£150. Branches in Bristol, Chel-
tenham and Exeter.

Green Shoes
**Station Road, Totnes, Devon TQ9 5HW
T 01803 864997**
Handmade boots, shoes and sandals
available in leather or vegan material. Can
be made to order for men, women and
children. Sizes infant 4 to child's 3, adults
2–14. Prices child's £26–£52; adult's
£42–£140. New designs each season and a
mail-order catalogue is available.

Omah Shoes
**4 Riverside Place, St James Street,
Taunton, Somerset TA1 1JH
T 01823 331435**
Omah sell all types of women's shoes,
sizes 36–42 (sizes 43 and 44 can be
obtained too). Prices £20–£100. There
is no mail-order service or catalogue
but Omah are happy to post shoes to
customers.

Soled Out
**Unit 8, Forge Lane, Moorlands Industrial
Estate, Saltash, Cornwall PL12 6LX
T 01752 841080**
Soled Out make men's, women's, children's and orthopaedic footwear, but
they love making one-offs too – Elvis
Boots and Bull Dog Boots to mention a
couple. Thus, as well as making comfortable or casual boots, shoes and sandals they will gladly create wacky shoes
in any size for 'theatrical' and 'party'
types. Sizes start at 5 for children and go
up to 16 1/2 for adults. Prices £30–£300.
Soled Out are happy for customers to

visit the workshop, as they say customer care is very important to them; goody bags for children are often made up. They serve the whole of the UK by mail order (catalogue available).

SUSSEX

Ideal Footwear
Chilgrove, Chichester,
West Sussex PO18 9HU
T 01243 535305

This company's motto is 'Problem Feet – No Problem'. They make to measure men's and women's shoes and boots for any occasion, including sports. Any size can be made, and all surgical needs can be met; styles can be copied from originals or clear illustrations. Prices £280–£400. There is a catalogue and although there is no mail-order service there are fitting rooms in Bath, Maidenhead, Tenterden and Chichester. Home visiting is also available.

Railton Ward
1–2 Nepcote Parade, Nepcote Lane,
Findon Village, West Sussex BN14 0SE
T 01903 873781

Ladies' narrow-fitting shoes. Sizes $3^{1}/_{2}$ to 10 in width fittings AA and B. Prices £40–£100.

Vegetarian Shoes
12 Gardner Street, Brighton,
East Sussex BN1 1UP
T 01273 691913   F 01273 679379

VS are dedicated to providing alternatives to leather. They have an enormous selection of shoes\available, such as trainers, Doc Martens, Birkenstocks, steel-toed and formal in quality breathable synthetics. Prices £30–£84. Sizes 3–12 (in some styles to 15). Ring for a free colour catalogue; will deliver to anywhere in the UK next day and within the week to the rest of the world.

YORKSHIRE

Kate Francis
The Old Stable, 812b Ecclesall Road,
Banner Cross, Sheffield S11 8TD
T 0114 268 2329

Kate Francis makes made-to-measure casual and walking shoes for men and women. Sizes $2–13^{1}/_{2}$ available to very wide fittings. Price range is £78–£115. They also make made-to-measure vegan alternatives to leather. Catalogue and mail-order service available.

Medissa
115 Queen Street, Morley,
Leeds LS27 8HE
T 0113 2530369

Medissa have all types of shoes (walking, sandals, formal) for women only. Sizes 8 to $12^{1}/_{2}$ in fittings AA, B, C, D, E, EE. They provide mail order and a catalogue and also do one-day events in the Midlands, Lancashire, Yorkshire, Tyneside, Birmingham, Humberside and Merseyside (call for details), as well as having the shop in Leeds. Prices £40–£65.

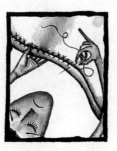

dressmakers

The following directory is a list of dressmakers near you and gives an idea of what they do, how much they charge, etc. None is particularly recommended by me; I haven't visited their premises or tried them out. They either wrote in when I asked for dressmakers to do so, or were recommended by readers. To protect yourself, it's always a good idea to ask to see examples of past work and perhaps talk to satisfied customers. Take time to discuss what you want and listen to what they have to say. I once insisted on having a structured dress made for me out of (lined) chiffon, and although the result was fantastic, it didn't have quite the uplift I had been hoping for. I'd be interested to have feedback on this section – very good or bad service needs to be brought to my attention, so in future editions I can make a note of recommendations to help other readers. A couturier dressmaker will be more expensive, but they will design an outfit for you and you will have the garment made first in calico toile so you can get an idea of how it will fit. These extra details cost but are worth it for special pieces. You must call for an appointment with these dressmakers before setting out.

EAST ANGLIA

Jane Leeburn
Tankerville House, 310 Norwich Road,
Ipswich, Suffolk IP1 4HD
T 01473 461982

Ladies' and children's wear. Price range: Dresses from £75 (adults), £45 (children); skirt/trousers from £45 (adults), £30 (children); jacket/coat from £100 (adults), £75 (children); waistcoats from £35. Prices include toile and fitting but not material. Time taken: from one week, depending on complexity. Notice period: one month approx. Areas covered: Suffolk and related areas – could be postal. Additional information: can use patterns or make up designs, but if pattern has to be made charges will be extra.

Liz McCullagh
Icknield, Coles Lane, Brinkley,
nr Newmarket, Suffolk CB8 0SD
T 01638 507 238

Bridal, evening dresses and ball gowns. Price range: bridal gowns from £300; evening dresses and bridesmaid dresses from £100; child's bridesmaid dresses from £60. Prices include design, pattern-making and fittings but not materials. Time taken: Bridal gowns, evening dresses and bridesmaid dresses six weeks. Notice period: varies.

Wedding Belles
90 Bures Road, Sudbury,
Suffolk CO10 0SE
T 01787 372285

Silk bridal gowns, bridesmaid dresses, mother-of-bride outfits, waistcoats, ties, etc. Price range: silk gowns from £400, including design, fabric, netting, etc. Time taken: Two months for wedding gowns. Notice period: wedding gowns three–four months; bridesmaid dresses two months. Additional information: an interview is arranged with bride and mother to discuss all aspects of the gown with the dressmaker and close contact is maintained throughout making of dress, with at least three fittings.

LONDON

Barber Green
Room 17, 33–35 St John's Square,
London EC1M 4DS
T 0171 608 0362

Clothes for executive ladies. Price range: jacket and skirts from £595, including fabric and lining; dresses from £295, including fabric; trousers from £150, including fabric. One fitting and then completion; 50 per cent deposit on order. Time taken: suit three weeks; skirts and dresses one week. Notice period: about a month, depending on time of year. Additional information: specialize in fitting unusual figures: very small to larger sizes (up to size 24). Alterations undertaken.

Christina Page
Battersea, London SW11
T 0171 924 5154 (by appointment only)

Bridal and special-occasion wear for women, bridesmaids, pageboys and groom's waistcoat. Price range: wedding dresses from £700, including fabric and toile; bridesmaid dresses from £150, inclusive; tailored silk or linen suits from £300. Time taken: wedding dresses two weeks; tailored suits one week. Notice period: at least two months. Additional information: a small collection is available to try on for style and fit, as well as a large range of fabrics to choose from.

Dawn Brewer Designs
Top Flat, 10 Stanley Gardens, London W11 2ND
T 0171 727 1916
Evening wear, bridal wear and special occasions. Price range: evening dresses from £400; wool jackets from £300. Prices include linings, fittings and toile but not material and buttons. Time taken: one week. Notice period: four–six weeks. Additional information: a wardrobe service is available and designer will attend weddings to assist the bride. There is a large stock of samples and fabric sourcing for clients can be done.

Diane Loney Hand Framed Knitwear
45/46 Charlotte Road, London EC2A 3PD
T 0171 613 1121 (and fax)
Specialist knitwear designer developing hand-crafted/hand-framed knitwear for ready to wear and evening wear. Price range: dresses from £250, separates from £150, accessories from £45. Time taken: jackets, trousers, shirts and dresses four weeks; skirts two weeks. Notice period: jackets, trousers, shirts and dresses four weeks; skirts two weeks.

Dressense
4 Hounslow Avenue, Hounslow, Middlesex TW3 2DX
T 0181 894 6573
Dresses, tailored suits and evening wear. Price range: dresses from £100; suits from £200. Time taken: two weeks for a suit. Notice period: two–three weeks, to include at least one fitting.

Heather Magoon
10 Rede Place, London W2 4TU
T 0171 221 7876
Model hats made to order or for hire or purchase from collection. Price range: made to order £50–£150, depending on materials and work involved. Hats for hire £25 + full price of hat as deposit. Additional information: will experiment with unusual styles, shapes and materials but does not make wide-brimmed Ascot wonders.

Imtaz Khaliq Couture Tailoring
37 South Molton Street, London W1Y 1HA (second floor)
T 0171 355 2202 (and fax)/0958 550816
Couture tailored suits for women only. Price range: skirt suit from £700; trouser suit £740; blouse £200; dress £440. Prices include fabric, fitting and toile. Every client has an individual pattern made. Time taken: four–six weeks, including initial consultation; can accommodate rush orders. Notice period: one week.

Joanna Bell
119 Nightingale Lane, London N8 7LG
T 0181 341 6459/0421 033258
Bridal and evening wear. Price range: wedding gowns £700–£1,200; evening gowns from £180; bridesmaids' gowns from £110. Prices include toile, fittings and material. Time taken: wedding gowns two months; evening gowns one month – depends on time of year. Notice period: wedding gowns minimum two months, but in July, August and September four months. Additional information: headdresses and veils are also made to complete the bridal outfit.

Joe Allen Design Consultants Ltd
20 Cross Street, London N1 2BG
T 0171 704 1013; fax: 0171 704 9532
Ladies and gents tailoring. Price range: gents' two-piece suits £450–£800; ladies' two-piece suits £300–£600; trousers £75–£125; shirts £50–£100; skirts £50–£100. These prices include consultations, fittings, toile but not fabric. Time taken: suits four weeks maximum; single garments one–two weeks. Notice period: five days, including fitting date; suits minimum two weeks. Additional infor-

mation: alteration and repair service available; buttonhole services; three-month tailoring and dressmaking courses for beginners and advanced.

June Taylor
Studio 3, The Mews, 46/52 Church Road, London SW13 0DQ
T 0181 563 1492
All aspects of ladieswear and men's shirts and waistcoats; tailored suits; ladies' occasional wear and bridal. Price range: from about £500 (without fabric) for a ladies' suit (skirt and jacket), which includes about three fittings. Time taken: three weeks. Notice period: one month from initial consultation. Additional information: aim is to achieve a perfect fit and complement the client's figure within the style they require using only the best fabrics, which can be supplied if required. Prices include a design consultation fee.

Lessin and Brown
42 Ambler Road, London N4 2QV
T 0171 359 2108 (and fax)
Bridal, special occasion wear, tailoring, embroidery, beading. Price range: wedding dresses from £700; women's suits from £400; cocktail dresses from £250. Prices include fabric, fittings, toile, etc. Time taken: from two weeks. Notice period: varies according to season.

Lily Jones
Abacus Business Centre, 30 Rugby Road, Twickenham, Middlesex TW1 1DG
T 0181 891 4346; F: 0181 891 6259
Costume-making for all occasions and all sizes: special occasions, weddings, theatre, fancy dress, party clothing for children, women and men. Also have stock for hire of vintage clothing and accessories in various sizes. Telephone for an appointment.

Qiana
The Business Village, Broomhill Road, London SW18 4JQ
T 0181 871 5076
Ladies' and men's tailoring, bridal, special-occasion wear, children's wear.

Price range: straight skirt £80; trousers £120; jackets £250–£350; day dresses from £250; bridal gowns from £800. Prices exclude fabric and trimmings. Notice period: book as early as possible but can accommodate rush orders. Additional information: Qiana pride themselves on making exact copies of client's favourite garment. Specialize in period costumes for television and films, and period bridal gowns.

Sarah Pinkster
25 Ewald Road, London SW6 3NB
T 0171 384 1601
Bridal wear, wedding and Ascot outfits, evening wear. Price range: wedding dresses from £850, including material, fittings and toile; evening dresses from £180 + material; bridesmaid and page outfits from £90 + material; waistcoats from £70 + material; suits from £200 + material. Time taken: wedding dress four fittings over eight weeks; bridesmaid and page one fitting; suits two fittings; evening wear two–three fittings. Notice period: bridal wear three–four months; suits and evening dresses one–two months. Additional information: daytime and early evening appointments are available Mon–Fri; all items are hand-finished.

MIDLANDS

Charlotte Walker
2 Hawthorne Terrace, Leek, Staffordshire, ST13 6AW
T 01538 371363
Ladies' wear: suits, evening, special-occasion and bridal wear. Price range: dresses from £95; skirts from £75; jackets from £180; evening wear from £180; trousers from £80; bridal gowns from £750. All prices include design, pattern-cutting, fittings, toile and materials. First consultation is free. Time taken: skirts, trousers and dresses one–two weeks; evening/special-occasion wear three–four weeks; bridal gowns six–eight weeks. Notice period: day wear two–four weeks; evening wear

four–eight weeks; bridal wear four–six months.

NORTH EAST

Frances Anderson
1 The Row, Longhoughton, Alnwick, Northumberland NE66 3AW
T 01665 577585
E-MAIL frances.anderson@onyxnet.co.uk
WEB SITE http://web.onyxnet.co.uk/
frances.anderson@onyxnet.co.uk
Hand-crafted clothing, knitwear and accessories for men and women. Patterns include hand-printing and dyeing. Choose from collection or commission own design. Special-occasion and bridal wear done by commission. Prices: accessories from £55 (e.g., felt hat), clothing from £150. Prices include fabric and toile. Time taken: from current collection six–eight weeks; special commissions six–eight weeks; bridal four–six months. Some styles and accessories in stock. Notice period: four–eight weeks from date of ordering; four–six months for bridal wear. Additional information: fabric is hand-dyed and/or printed and can be done to taste. Accessories will be made to fit a specific theme.

MCM

14 Victoria Avenue, Barnsley S70 2BH
T Lorraine McClellan on 01132 824690 or June Meade on 01226 205316
Ladies' wear. Price range: ladies' jackets from £175; trousers/skirts from £100; shirts/tops from £80; dresses £125. Time taken: two–four weeks, depending on fitting and design. Notice period: one month, depending on fabric requested; two weeks if stock fabric. Additional information: understated classics for all sizes, using only quality fabrics – woven cashmere, wool crêpe, silks, linens, etc.

SCOTLAND

Angus and Hamie Hats
c/o Claire Tester (Milliner),
Kinkell Bridge, By Auchterarder,
Perthshire, PH3 1LD
T 01764 663335
Traditionally hand-blocked and hand-sewn felt, straw and covered hats made to measure. Price range: ready-to-wear straw hats from £50; special occasion (e.g. Ascot) from £100; prices includes initial consultation, measurement and fitting. Time taken: minimum one week, maximum three weeks. Notice period: four–eight weeks usually. Additional information: designer hats to modest numbers. Original and elegant designs made to match client's outfit or whim.

McCance–Glasgow (Clothes for Women)
6a Manse Road, Bearsden,
Glasgow G61 3PT
T 0141 942 2373
Modern clothes for women by designer/manufacturer. Finest-quality fabrics, simple shapes, clean lines. Made to measure is available from the collection or by commissioned design. Bridal wear by commissioned design only. Price range: evening dresses from £300; lined jackets from £500; lined skirts from £180; wool jersey suit (unlined) from £450. Prices include fabric and two–three fittings as necessary. Time taken: minimum two weeks. Notice period: variable. Additional information: All designs are exclusive to McCance–Glasgow and an extensive choice of fabric is available. They also offer a shopping service for accessories to complete an outfit, which costs £20 per hour plus travel costs.

SOUTH EAST

Caterina and Carmelina Couture Dressmakers
311 Iffley Road, Oxford OX4 4AG
T 01865 723905 (by appointment only)
Bridal wear, mother of bride, all attendants, grooms' waistcoats, veils, headdresses. Special-occasion and evening wear. Price range: from £600, including fitting and toile, for bridal. Fabric can be selected from wide range of silk samples or provided by client. Time taken: two–three months. Notice period:

two–six months. Additional information: will do alterations; appointments can be made for evening and weekends to suit client. Portfolio of previous work available for viewing.

Jill Sanders Exclusive Dressmaker
Bramley Cottage, 9 Vicarage Hill, Hartley Wintney, Hants RG27 8EH
T 01252 842314

Bridal and special occasion wear. Price range: wedding dress from £400; executive business wear; suit with two skirts from £300. Prices include fittings, toile, making up and haberdashery, but not fabric. Time taken: bridal wear up to three months; other garments depends on workload and availability of clients for fittings. Notice period: three months. Additional information: can offer a wardrobe extension and co-ordination programme; patterns can be made from favourite clothes and will restyle existing clothes.

Olney Originals
Olney House, High Street, Olney, Bucks MK46 6EB
T 01234 241440

Olney concentrate mostly on wedding dresses, evening dresses, mother-of-bride, bridesmaid and pageboy outfits. Price range: from £500 for wedding dresses. Time taken: wedding dresses eight weeks; others six weeks. Notice period: variable. Additional information: Olney also come to London to meet clients, at the Parrot Club, Basil Street Hotel, Basil Street, SW3.

Rachel Barran
St Helens, Bay Road, Freshwater Bay, Isle of Wight PO40 9QS
T 01983 752336 (and fax)

Dressmaking and ladies' tailoring. Price range: ladies' lined jacket £60; summer dresses from £40; lined wool dresses from £60; lined kick-pleat skirt from £35; summer skirts from £25; sleeveless tops from £20; blouses from £25. Prices do not include materials. Time taken: four weeks; can be less if for specific

date. Notice period: none. Additional information: can copy existing garments and make alterations. Also makes curtains.

SOUTH WEST

Annabel Ayres
Sheephouse Farm, Warleigh, Bath BA1 8EE
T 01225 852487

Bridal, day and evening wear. Price range: wedding dresses from £300; suits from £175. Prices include toile and fittings but not fabrics. Time taken: four–five fittings for wedding dresses. Notice period: depends on workload. Additional information: all garments are specifically designed and made for the individual.

Dawn Brewer Designs
Orchardleigh, Broadhempston, Nr Totnes, Devon TQ9 6BQ
T 01803 8123444

Evening wear, bridal wear and special occasions. Price range: evening dresses from £400; wool jackets from £300. Prices include linings, fittings and toile but not material and buttons. Time taken: one week. Notice period: four–six weeks. Additional information: a wardrobe service is available and designer will attend weddings to assist the bride. There is a large stock of samples and fabric sourcing for clients can be done. [DBD also work from a London address – see 'London' section.]

Heather Martin
– Hand-decorated Clothing
Yew Tree House, Cliff Road, Sherston, Wiltshire SN16 0LN
T 01666 840375

Special-occasion wear decorated with hand or machine embroidery, appliqué, beading. Style of garment and design of decoration discussed with client to ensure a one-off creation. Price range: velvet embroidered jacket £250–£400, including fabric and fittings. Machine embroidery for wedding dresses £200–£300, exclusive of fabric and making of dress. Time taken: jacket three–four weeks. Notice period: one–two months. Additional information: works in association with Sue Palmer – designer dressmaker – who also specializes in suits, jackets and alternative wedding outfits (T 01666 840486).

Sheila Brough Designer Dressmaker
Thimble Cottage, 1 Jamaica Terrace,
Heamoor, Penzance,
Cornwall TR18 3HQ
T 01736 366605

Bridal, mother-of-bride, evening wear, special-occasion wear (women's). Price range: bridal gowns from £450; other designs from £175. Prices include fittings, materials and toile. Time taken: three weeks minimum. Notice period: bridal gowns six months minimum; evening wear two months; mother-of-bride three months – always heavily booked during summer season. Additional information: individually designed garments and wide range of fabrics available, including hand-painted, beaded and embroidered fabrics created by the designer.

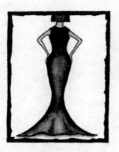

size 16 plus

I think of this as the most important directory in a way, because it covers what interests so many since so few 'do' size 16 and above clothes. It lists those that do – chain stores, specialist individuals and catalogues . . . whoever takes an interest in larger clothes. Some go up to very impressive sizes, others not so much. All have been recommended by readers. Any further comments to add, please write in. The first section, 'Nationwide', covers chain stores, mail order or labels that don't have their own retail outlet but sell to stores *nationwide*. Remember to look in the 'Underwear' and 'Swimwear' directories too, as they also cover 16 plus.

Anna Scholz

T 0181 964 3040 for your nearest stockist
Contemporary designer of womenswear.
Size range: 10–28. Price range: £60–£600
for a winter coat. Twenty stockists,
including Selfridges and Harrods.

Classic Combination Catalogue

53 Dale Street, Manchester M60 6ES
T 0800 262 717 (quoting CLA2499)
Classic Combination is a catalogue company which carried out a sizing survey
five years ago which found that the
British Standard Sizes set in the 1950s
were outdated because the size and shape
of women had changed. Their range,
which includes smart suits, casual clothes,
separates, evening wear, underwear and
nightwear, was designed to suit women's
bodies in the 1990s. Size range: 12–26.
Price range: £10–£70. Catalogue ordering
on above number.

Dans-Ez Plus

T 01843 866300 for stockists/mail order
Aerobic wear for 16 plus sizes available
from sportswear departments and by
mail order. Two ranges available: a ballet
range, which has been going for twenty-
five years, and an active-wear range,
including leotards, leggings and the
'minimal bounce' aerobic bra. Size
range: 16–20. Price range: from £23.49
for leggings. Catalogue available from
above number.

Elvi

**T 0121 212 2392; seventy-one shops and
department-store concessions**
In-house-designed co-ordinated range
of clothing from coats through to jackets, skirts, dresses, trousers, blouses,
swimwear, accessories and nightwear.
Specially trained staff can give advice on
shape and fit for the larger customer.
Customer service through Birmingham
office (0121 212 2392). Brochure and
branch list available. Alteration service
available in all outlets. Loyalty card
offering discount on future purchases.
Size range: 14–26. Price range: jackets
£90; skirts £50; blouses £45. Opening
hours depend on local branch.

Evans

T 0800 7318287 for customer services
Well-fitting, comfortable clothes across
a broad range of styles from formal to
casual. Size range: 16–30, with selected
lines in 30/32. Price range: approx.
£30–£95, with dresses £30–£70. There is
a made-to-measure service available at
the Regent Street store (enquiries: 0171
927 3960). The range of styles for this
service is different to the styles available
in the stores. Prices vary depending on
cloth type and style, but approx.
£250–£350 for a jacket and £120 for
trousers/skirt. It takes two–three weeks.
The 'Evans Direct' catalogue comes out
every three months and offers mail
order mainly of styles that are available
in the shops, with some exclusive lines
(order line: 0990 991111).

Fashion World Catalogue

53 Dale Street, Manchester M60 6ES
T 0800 262 717 (quoting FW2499)
This mail-order range specializes in

good-value fashion for sizes 12–26.
Smart suits, casual wear, comfortable
tops, trousers and skirts, evening wear,
underwear and nightwear are all available. Over 300 items cost under £20.
Price range: £10–£70. For a complimentary catalogue, call the above number.

Fifty Plus Catalogue
53 Dale Street, Manchester M60 6ES
T 0800 262 717 (quoting FPS2491)

This mail-order company is aimed at the
over-fifties. A wide selection of garments, including smart, casual, evening
wear and underwear, is available, all in
sizes 12–26. Price range: £10–£100. For a
complimentary catalogue, call the above
number.

Higginbotham Traditional Nightwear
PO Box 121, Diss, Norfolk IP21 4JN
T 01379 668833; fax: 01379 668844
E-MAIL
nightwear@higginbotham.demon.co.uk

Higginbotham is a mail-order company
selling nightshirts, dressing gowns,
kimonos and pyjamas for men and
women. A free colour brochure is available on request. Orders dispatched on
the same day by first-class post (90 per
cent arrive next day). Usually every item
is available. All garments are made from
finest cotton poplin and available in a
choice of traditional stripes. Attention
to detail includes self-fabric drawstring
waists, total piping, hang-up loops, deep
pockets. All garments are extremely
generously cut, so bear this in mind
when ordering. Size range: nightshirts
10–22; pyjamas 10–18; gowns 10–22;
men's 34"–53" chest. Price range:
£45–£75.

House of Fraser
T 0171 963 2236; stores nationwide

House of Fraser's own label has recently
been rejuvenated. Lots of other plus-
sized labels are also sold. Size range:
18–26. Prices start at £20 for HoF's own
label. Personal shopping is available free
in some branches; call for details. Opening hours vary, so contact local store.

Index Extra
T 0800 401080 mail order

The 'Style Unlimited' collection in the
catalogue is a range which covers sizes
12–26. Shirt prices start at £20, skirts at
£25. Order lines open from 7 a.m.–11
p.m., seven days a week.

Long Tall Sally
T 0181 649 9009; twenty-five branches
nationwide

A full range of clothes for tall women
over 5'9": e.g., coats, jeans, suits, dresses
and swimwear. Specialists in tall
women's fashion. Everything repropor-
tioned for women over 5'9". Free mail-
order catalogue six times a year.
Exclusive range; largest selection of
clothes for tall women in the UK. Size
range: 10–22. Price range: jeans, blouses
and dresses from £29.95; skirts from
£26.95; coats from £82.95. Opening
hours vary from store to store. Mail
order open on Sundays (0181 649 9009).

Marks & Spencer
T 0171 935 4422 for your nearest branch

The mighty M&S do tailoring, casual
wear lingerie, sports and swimwear in
sizes 8–20. Prices vary but all good
value. Opening hours are according to
individual store.

Rogers + Rogers
T 01923 474400 for your nearest stockist

Rogers + Rogers was established in 1992
by Jeffrey Rogers. The collection features
colours and shapes from the JR range
translated into larger sizes. Alongside
basic pieces there are also interpretations
of seasonal trends. Size range: 16–24.
Price range: £9.99–£125.

Shapely Figures Catalogue
53 Dale Street, Manchester M60 6ES
T 0800 262717
(quoting ref number AWL 2499)

A forty-eight-page lingerie and nightwear catalogue filled to the brim with
all-in-ones, bras, knickers, camisoles and
nightwear up to a size 54G. Prices start
at £9.99 for a pack of two bras. Call the
above number for a catalogue.

TAILLISSIME
T 0500 777 777 for mail order
A French mail-order catalogue specializing in tall and large sizes for men and women. Prices start at around £17.99 for a T-shirt. Clothes are available in a wide range of lengths and sizes. Size range: for women 14–30, with trousers available in three different leg lengths; for men chest sizes are approx. 40"–55", waists 36"–55". The catalogue is free on the above number and lines are open 8 a.m.–11 p.m., seven days a week.

EAST ANGLIA

Blake House
2a Earsham Street, Bungay,
Suffolk NR35 1AG
T 01986 893131
Blake House stocks suits, dresses, trousers, etc. by labels such as Finn Karelia, Quimo and Norman Linton. They are happy to send garments on approval and promise a personal service. Size range: 14–34. Price range: £9.99–£60 for a top; £46–£200 for a suit. The shop is open daily 9 a.m.–5 p.m. (except Wed and Sun), and at any other time by appointment.

LONDON

Base
55 Monmouth Street, London WC2H 9DG
T 0171 240 8914
Day wear and accessories (e.g., belts) for women in sizes 16–28. Stock is very seasonal and is changed every eight–ten weeks. No mail-order service but they do work closely with loyal customers and will send out goods to them. Price range: from £70 for a skirt; from £150 for a jacket. Open 10 a.m.–6 p.m., Mon–Sat.

French and Teague
69 Gloucester Avenue, London NW1 8LD
T 0171 483 0733
Casual and dressy clothes in luxurious fabrics. Size range: 16–32. Price range: from £180. French and Teague is stocked in Liberty, Harrods and Self-ridges, as well as at the Gloucester Avenue address. The range is also stocked at Women at Large in Coventry [see separate entry in 'Midlands' section]. Staff at the Gloucester Avenue shop are happy to discuss what's available over the phone with customers from outside London, and will send swatches of fabric when possible. The shop is open 10 a.m.–6 p.m., Mon–Sat.

Harrington Supersizes Ltd
129 The Broadway, London NW7 4RN
T 0181 959 2312
Harrington specializes in occasion wear but also stocks day wear. Size range: 16–34. Price range: trousers from £75; evening dresses £150–£550. Open 9 a.m.–5.30 p.m., Mon–Sat, and 10 a.m.–2 p.m., Sun.

Harrods
Knightsbridge, London SW1X 7XL
T 0171 730 1234
Plus Collections is situated on the first floor and stocks designer wear for women, including career, occasion and casual wear. The department has many exclusive ranges from around the world. Staff are knowledgeable and provide individual service. Size range: 18–26. Price range: £60–£500. Open 10 a.m.–6 p.m., Mon, Tues, Sat; 10 a.m.–7 p.m., Wed, Thur, Fri.

John Neville
5 Club Row, London E1 6JX
T 0171 739 8936
Designer clothes for all occasions, including day, evening and occasion wear, in many fabrics. Size range: 16–34. Price range: £50–£200. Requirements, patterns and sketches can be discussed and sent by post if necessary. The studio is open 9 a.m.–4 p.m., Mon–Fri, and on Sat morning by arrangement.

Ken Smith Designs
6 Charlotte Place, London W1P 1AQ
T 0171 631 3341
Known for special-occasion wear, also stocks ladies' casual and tailored

separates. Although there is no catalogue, they often send out 'goody
parcels' on approval for people to look
at anywhere in the UK. Size range:
18/20–30+. Price range: from £69 for
summer trousers. Open 10 a.m.–6 p.m.,
weekdays, 10 a.m.–2 p.m., Sat.

Rita Jarvis
16 Queen's Grove, London NW8 6EL
T 0171 722 1127
Rita makes simple, stylish clothes in
cottons, silks and velvets. All clothes
are individually made so any size can be
catered for. Price range: £36–£150. An
appointment is necessary as Rita works
from home, but she does have an open
day on the first Saturday of each month
from noon. Telephone the above number for more information or a small
mail-order catalogue.

Sixteen 47
69 Gloucester Avenue, London NW1 8LD
T 0171 483 0733
As the shop name suggests, sizes here
range from 16–47. Affordable separates,
including evening wear, in good-quality
fabrics with prices starting at £45. Like
its sister shop, French and Teague [see
above], staff are happy to advise customers over the phone and send out
swatches of fabric when they can. Open
10 a.m.–6 p.m., Mon–Sat.

MIDLANDS

Woman at Large
2 Spon Street, Coventry CV1 3BA
T 01203 550300
Good selection of casual, day wear,
business wear, evening wear and special-occasion wear – quality clothes in
larger sizes. Large fitting rooms and no
assistants below a size 16. Housed in a
stunning medieval building and many
people travel long distances to visit.
Size range: 16–30 (on occasion they
can also get 30+). Price range: from £40
for a skirt or blouse to £600 for a top-
of-the-range wedding outfit. Open
9.30 a.m.–5 p.m., Mon–Sat.

YORKSHIRE

Sundial
5 Lendal, York YO1 2AQ
T 01904 644 410
Co-ordinates, separates, smarter casual
wear, plus a small collection of cocktail
wear, coats and rainwear. Sundial say
they are York's only independent boutique specializing in larger-size fashion. Wheelchair access and personal
service. Principal ranges stocked
include Finn Karelia, Lucia, Almia and
Toddy. Size range: 18–28. Price range:
£40–£250. Open 9.30 a.m.–5 p.m.,
Mon–Sat.

SCOTLAND

Cocoon Coats
Lomond Industrial Estate, Alexandria,
Dunbarton G83 0TL
T 01389 755511
Cocoon Coats are available mail order
(catalogue available) or from one of
their three shops in Alexandria, Edinburgh and London – ring above number for addresses. They sell only coats
and matching rain hats, but all are
made to suit any size or height. They
do have some coats in stock but most
are made to order. Size range: 8–30.
All coats are machine-washable. Price
range: £155–£250. The shops in London and Edinburgh are open 10
a.m.–5 p.m., six days a week, and the
Alexandria shop is open 9 a.m.–5
p.m., Mon–Fri, and 11 a.m.–5 p.m.,
Sat–Sun.

SOUTH WEST

That New Shop
44 Parsonage Street, Dursley,
Glos GL11 4AD
T 01453 546832
6 High Street, Malmesbury,
Wilts SN16 9AL
T 01666 825 098
That New Shop say of themselves: 'We
dress from ages 18–80 in clothes that
take you from Waitrose to work to

weddings. Shapes are more flowingly female than tightly tailored. Our larger sizes get you noticed for the right reasons. Definitely no glitz or "Mother of the bride".' They hold twice-yearly informal fashion shows in their Dursley branch (offering a 10 per cent discount) for mailing-list customers – the first 100 replies get in. Size range: 10–20. Price range: dresses £60–£150; jackets £100–£150; skirts £50–£100; knitwear £40–£100; trousers £40–£75. Open 9.30 a.m.–5.30 p.m., Mon–Fri, 9.30 a.m.–5 p.m., Sat.

Vivace!
2 Bridge Street, Richmond-upon-Thames, Surrey TW9 1TQ
T 0181 948 7840
Vivace! have been established for eight years and aim to provide women with a range of casual wear through to evening wear. Emphasis is on the combination of fabric and colour with directional design. The style of clothes is aimed at women from their thirties to their fifties who have a very extensive business and social life. Size range: 16–22. Price range: £20 for a T-shirt; jacket, shirt and skirt £265–£325; and £350 for a ball gown. Customers are kept up to date on stock with regular newsletters. Open 10 a.m.–5.30 p.m., Mon–Fri, 10 a.m.–6 p.m., Sat.

SUSSEX

Emma Plus
16 Church Street, Brighton, East Sussex BN1 1RB
T 01273 327240
Emma Plus specialize in clothes sized 18–34. Casual wear, suiting, evening wear, lingerie and swimwear all available. Price range: £30 for a blouse; £300 for evening wear. Solar swimwear (and accessories) are stocked in sizes 20–30, though not all year round. A range of underwear is available, with bras sized from 38B–48FF, priced from £17. Very friendly customer service. Open 10 a.m.–5.30 p.m., Tues–Sat.

Inside Out Designs
34 Upper St James's Street, Kemptown, Brighton, East Sussex BN2 1JN
T 01273 674819
Clothes are individual, comfortable and well made. Colour is a major feature and changes from season to season. Main lines include adjustable skirts, tops, trousers, jackets and dresses. All in natural fabrics. Some hand-woven, others hand-painted. The designer is a slightly eccentric size 16, and aware of arms, tums and the need for pockets! The clothes are available from selected stockists, their friendly shop in Brighton, or by Visa telephone transaction. A simple line-drawing catalogue, with swatches of fabric, is also available. Size range: 10–22. Price range: £35–£75. Open 9.30 a.m.–5.30 p.m., Mon–Sat (closed Wed).

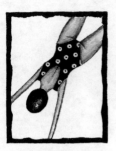

swimwear

This directory came about because so many people wanted to know who sold swimwear bits separately: e.g., where you could buy a size 12 bottom with a size 16 top. So here is a round-up of just about every swimwear manufacturer, with sizes, prices and enquiry numbers; 'separates' means they sell tops and bottoms separately. This directory also covers men's swimwear.

Anna Club by La Perla
Sophisticated swimwear aimed at the older customer; quality fabrics and exotic prints.
Sizes: 8–18
Prices: from £140
Enquiries: 0171 436 5864
Separates: yes, on some lines

Aquasuit by La Perla
A very versatile range from La Perla; lots of prints and less expensive than other La Perla lines.
Sizes: 8–20 in some styles
Prices: from £80
Enquiries: 0171 436 5864
Separates: yes, on some lines

Arena
European performance swimwear using advanced technology and fabrics developed for comfort and durability.
Sizes: 28"–42"chest for women; 30"–40" waist for men
Prices: £16.99–£34.99 for women; £9.99–£14.99 for men
Enquiries: 01524 8487878
Separates: no

Armand Basi
Men's and women's sporty swimwear from Barcelona.
Sizes: S, M and L
Prices: £40–£100
Enquiries: 0171 349 5859
Separates: no

Bhs
A sporty range, including a choice of underwired or cropped tops and different leg lines.
Sizes: 10–20
Prices: £10 per piece
Enquiries: 0171 262 3288
Separates: yes

Björn Borg
Sporty range which varies according to fashions; also available mail order.
Sizes: S–XL
Prices: £40 upwards
Enquiries: 0171 937 2226
Separates: yes

Bravissimo
Mail-order cupped swimwear catering for large cup sizes.
Sizes: 30C–44HH
Prices: £40–£50
Enquiries: 07000 2442727
Separates: not at time of going to press, but under review

Bust Stop
Mail-order swimwear and bikinis catering for large cup sizes; also a shop in Middlesex.
Sizes: 32–40, C–FF cup (though not in all styles)
Prices: £45–£60
Enquiries: 0181 943 9733
Separates: yes

Chanel
Designer swimwear and bikinis.
Sizes: 8–14
Prices: from £250
Enquiries: 0171 493 5040
Separates: no

Elle Active
Sporty, simple styling.

Sizes: 10–14
Prices: £15–£25 for bottoms; £25–£35
for tops; £30–£45 for swimsuits
Enquiries: 0171 436 0222
Separates: yes

Elvi
All-in-one pieces with built-in bust sup-
port.
Sizes: 16–26 (approx. 36C–42C)
Prices: £30–£40
Enquiries: 0121 212 2392
Separates: no

Fantasie
Cup-sized swimwear, longer length and
tummy panels; post-mastectomy catered
for. As well as separates, a choice of bot-
toms is available in addition to bikini
pants: thongs, shorts or skirts.
Sizes: 32–44, B–G
Prices: £35–£70
Enquiries: 01536 760282
Separates: yes

Footprints
A range by Fanatsie aimed at the
younger customer.
Sizes: 30–38, A–FF
Prices: £40–£50
Enquiries: 01536 760282
Separates: yes

French Connection
Range of about ten styles (swimsuits and
bikinis) made up in different fabrics
available in summer; also available mail
order.
Sizes: S, M and L
Prices: £25–£35
Enquiries: 0171 399 7200
Separates: no

Gottex
Pareos, skirts and dresses to match
swimwear.
Sizes: 10–22 in some ranges
Prices: £100–£130 swimsuits; £85–£115
bikinis
Enquiries: 0171 584 2427
Separates: no

Harrods
Over twenty-five different brands
stocked in body, beach and swimwear
on first floor.
Sizes: 8–14
Prices: £9.95 (swim hats) to £400
Enquiries: 0171 730 1234
Separates: no

Hugo Boss
Men's fashionable and sporty trunks
and shorts.
Sizes: S, M and L
Prices: £25–£69
Enquiries: 0171 589 5522
Separates: no

Index Extra
Large range, some with tummy-control
panels, designed to be mixed and
matched; available mail order. Different
leg lengths available.
Sizes: 8–24 (selected lines)
Prices: from £18; £23 average swimsuit
Enquiries: 0345 979797 for a catalogue
Separates: yes

Joelynian
Cutting-edge women's swimwear, some
100 per cent UV-proof.
Sizes: 8–12
Prices: £60 for a bikini
Enquiries: 0171 267 4770
Separates: no

John Lewis
Brands stocked include Morgan, Vicido-
mini, Huit, Slix, Fantasie, Elle, Cos-
mopolitan, Too Hot Brazil, Jantzen and
Manuel Canovas and Armani at Peter
Jones only. Within Aquatics (JL own
brand) the Combini is a range of sepa-
rates with three styles of tops and three
styles of bottoms available.
Sizes: up to FF cup in some ranges
Prices: from £11.50 each item in the
Combini range
Enquiries: 0171 629 7711
Separates: yes

Knickerbox
Simply styled high-fashion swimwear
range in prints and plain colours.

Sizes: 8–16
Prices: £25–£45 bikini sets; underwired bikini tops from £16 and bottoms from £10; swimsuits £25–£45.
Enquiries: 0171 284 1744
Separates: yes

La Perla Mare
Cruisewear led by the latest fashions, with great visual appeal.
Sizes: 8–16
Prices: from £165
Enquiries: 0171 436 5864
Separates: yes, on some lines

La Perla Sport
Functional swimwear with sporty styling using high-quality Lycra fabrics.
Sizes: 8–16
Prices: from £130
Enquiries: 0171 436 5864
Separates: yes, on some lines

Lingerie Brazil
Flamboyant swimwear in bright colours.
Sizes: S, M and L
Prices: from £35
Enquiries: 0171 386 7062
Separates: no

Long Tall Sally
Long-line swimsuits.
Sizes: 12–20
Prices: £19.95–£29.95
Enquiries: 0181 649 9009
Separates: no

Malizia Mare
Diffusion range from La Perla; modern feminine styling.
Sizes: 8–16
Prices: from £90 for swimwear; co-ordinates may be less
Enquiries: 0171 436 5864
Separates: yes, on some lines; differs each season

Margaret Ann
A confidential and discreet service by appointment only; can cater for any size. Mastectomy swimwear available with pockets, and pockets can be fitted into client's own swimwear for a small charge. Margaret Ann is the holder of a 'Dear Annie' gold star [see p. 199].
Sizes: 30–50, B–G (30–38G only)
Prices: from £50
Enquiries: 01985 840520
Separates: no

Maru
Active sports swimwear with the latest fabric technology and a strong commitment to fit.
Sizes: 26"–40" (42" and 44" in selected lines); children's sizes 24"–32"
Prices: £19.95–£29.95 (men's from £9.95)
Enquiries: 01159 851212
Separates: no

Marvel Mare
The most raunchy of the La Perla swimwear lines, originally developed as lingerie; very colourful, with high cutting.
Sizes: 8–16
Prices: from £100
Enquiries: 0171 436 5864
Separates: yes, on some lines; differs each season

Nicole Farhi 'Swim'
Simple, streamlined pieces for men and women in keeping with the mainline collection.
Sizes: 8–14 women; S, M and L men
Prices: £79 average
Enquiries: 0171 499 8368
Separates: no

Oceano by La Perla
Sporty beachwear, simple styling, sleek lines and innovative fabrics.
Sizes: 8–16
Prices: from £110
Enquiries: 0171 436 5864
Separates: yes, on some lines; differs each season

Racing Green
Simple, styled classic mail-order swimwear in basic colours.
Sizes: 8–18, B and C
Prices: from £15 for a bikini halter top; from £25 for a swimsuit
Enquiries: 0990 411 111
Separates: yes

Rigby and Peller

Cup-sized swimwear from this famous underwear specialist. Brands include Fantasie, Gottex, Anna Club, Lidea, La Perla, Gideon Oberson. Mastectomy swimwear is available and pockets can be sewn into swimwear for £25 per pocket.
Sizes: 30–40, B–G
Prices: £50–£220
Enquiries: 0171 491 2200
Separates: no

Sam de Teran

String bikinis, halter-necks and under-wired glamorous swimwear often with sequins, frills and gingham. Bikinis can be mixed and matched.
Sizes: 10–16
Prices: bikini tops and bottoms start from £55; swimsuits from £105
Enquiries: 0171 584 0902
Separates: yes

Selfridges

Range includes Triumph, Fantasie, Calvin Klein, Sam de Teran, Armani, Gottex, La Perla, Dolce and Gabbana, Moschino and Jantzen.
Sizes: 10–24, some up to FF cup (depends on the brand)
Prices: £29 upwards
Enquiries: 0171 629 1234
Separates: no

Slix

Swimsuits and bikinis with cup sizes and tummy-control panels.
Sizes: 8–24, B–DD
Prices: £35–£65
Enquiries: 0181 450 3066
Separates: no

Speedo

Competition, training and leisure. Four leg lengths available: high, low, medium and classic
Sizes: 32"–42" on most
Prices: £10.99–£79.99
Enquiries: 0115 916 7000
Separates: no

Splash Out

Swimwear made to order at reasonable prices. All garments available in a longer length body; leg lines can be cut higher or lower according to specifications. Post-mastectomy swimwear, a range aimed at larger sizes and men's swimwear also available.
Sizes: to order; cup sizes up to F/G
Price: Swimsuits £25–£40; bikinis £12–£16 per piece
Enquiries: 01903 230861
Separates: yes

Taillissime

A wide choice of one-piece and two-piece comfortable swimwear in larger sizes available mail order.
Sizes: 14–30, A–E cup (not all sizes)
Prices: underwired bikinis from £18.50; swimsuits from £24.99
Enquiries: 0500 777777
Separates: yes

Triumph

Exceptionally well-fitting swimwear for all ages in contemporary styling, with the emphasis on cup sizing.
Sizes: 32A–48E, depending on style
Prices: £19–£65
Enquiries: 01793 720330
Separates: it depends on the retailer

Tweka

Beach and high-performance wear; also mastectomy suits, maternity wear, long-torso fittings, chlorine-resistant and tummy-control panels. Men's and children's also available.
Sizes: swimsuits 8–24, B–D, and bikinis 8–18, B–D; men's 30"–40" waist; children age 1–14
Prices: swimsuits £25–£60; bikinis £43–£48
Enquiries: 01702 436002
Separates: no

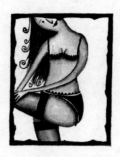

underwear

Agent Provocateur

Shops in Knightsbridge and Soho and mail order. Individual, sexy but never 'trashy' underwear and accessories. Twice-yearly collection; lots of corsetry and marabou.
Sizes: 32A–38F (can do special orders)
Prices: £35–£500
Enquiries: 0171 253 5123/mail order 01483 204469

Aubade

Upmarket fashion-oriented range, updated every six months.
Sizes: 32A–38E
Prices: bras £45–£60; knickers from £27
Enquiries: 01908 223003

Avon Cosmetics

Embrace is exclusive to Avon but they offer other brands too. Sports, lace, seamless, vests, knickers and glamorous, comfortable underwear for larger sizes available mail order or through local Avon representative.
Sizes: 32AA–46DD, though not in every style
Prices: from £6 for a bra
Enquiries: 0845 6050400

Axfords

Over twenty different styles of laced and boned corsets based on traditional patterns available mail order; catalogue £10.
Sizes: 18"–40" waists
Prices: from £50 up to £250 for leather corsets
Enquiries: 01273 327944; fax: 01273 220680; e-mail: axfords@axfords.com and website: http//www.axfords.com

Berlei

Bras include minimizers, maternity, 'Ultimate Comfort', 'Shock Absorber' (sports range made from cool max – a fabric which draws moisture away from the skin) and the 'Answers' range (strapless, backless and multi-way bras), as well as lacy ranges.
Sizes: 30AA–40G (not in everything); briefs S–XXL
Prices: £15–£25
Enquiries: 01525 850088

Björn Borg

Innovative and sporty cotton knickers, shorts, hip briefs, bras without fitted cups; appeals to younger customer, though becoming more sophisticated. Also available mail order.
Sizes: XS–L
Prices: £9.95–£50
Enquiries: 0171 937 2226

Bravissimo

A wide range of mail-order lingerie with emphasis on fuller cup sizes rather than large back sizes. Black, white, natural and ivory colours, as well as lots of colours available.
Sizes: 30C–44HH (focus on C–HH cup)
Prices: £20 for a bra; luxury ranges from £50
Enquiries: 0181 742 7593

Bust Stop

Mail-order catalogue (and one shop in Middlesex) specializing in smaller back and larger cup sizes. Brands include Fantasie, Silhouette, Rigby and Peller, Charnos, Ballet, Dans-ez, Exquisite

Form, Goddess, Berlei, Bravado, Braza, Sloggi and Triumph. All types of bras and bustiers stocked, as well as stockings and knickers.
Sizes: 30C–50I cup in some cases
Prices: Bras from £17
Enquiries: 0181 943 9733

Cacharal

A pretty, delicate range from Playtex with lots of lace and embroidery. Cotton, Tactel and Lycra bras and knickers.
Sizes: 32A–38D
Prices: Briefs from £8; bras from £15
Enquiries: 0500 362430

Carnival

American basques, strapless and low-back bras and knickers. Specializes in wedding lingerie. Catalogue costs £5, which is refundable against purchases.
Sizes: 32A–42DD
Prices: £22–£55
Enquiries: 0171 636 8129

Charnos

Glamorous and everyday pieces, including basques, bras, briefs, suspenders and wedding lingerie. High-fashion ranges with lots of sheer and lace fabrics and the 'Superfit' range, which includes their best-selling mini-mizer bra.
Sizes: 32A–38G in the classic ranges
Prices: From £11 for briefs; £45 for bras/basques
Enquiries: 0115 932 2191

Cosmopolitan

Three ranges licensed from the magazine for Cosmo women. 'Essentials' is very sporty, in black and white cotton with Lycra; 'Active' is black and white and lacy; 'Style' is quite vampish.
Sizes: 10–12, 14–16
Price: from £8 for a thong up to £40
Enquiries: 0116 246 0240

Dans-ez Plus

Sports bras without hooks, wires, darts or seams, and all-in-ones. The 'Minimal Bounce Bra', worn by famous sports stars, and also the 'Cross Training' bra.

Available in sixteen different colours.
Sizes: 32A–42E
Prices: From £22.99
Enquiries: 01843 866300 for nearest stockist and free catalogue

Fantasie

Bras and co-ordinated lingerie for the fuller-busted figure; also foundation wear, including corselets.
Sizes: 30–44, A–HH (not in every style); foundation wear 34"–42"; corset pants sized 25"–42"
Prices: from £7 for thongs; from £23 for bras; from £49 for girdles
Enquiries: 01536 760282

Fenwick

Fashion and basic underwear. Brands include Lejaby, Malizia, Chantelle, Hanro, Aubade, Marie Jo, Gossard, Warners, Passionata, Triumph, Rigby and Peller, Dior. Some lines may differ in different branches.
Sizes: 32AA–38GG
Prices: bras £11–£95
Enquiries: 0171 629 9161; mail order available from the Bond Street branch

Goddess

Bras, long-line bras to the waist and basques to the hips; specializes in larger sizes. Catalogue available for bridal wear.
Sizes: 32B–52F (basques) and up to 52H
Prices: from £35 for bras; from £70 for basques
Enquiries: 0171 636 8129

Gossard

Fashion-led, with emphasis on comfort and fabrics.
Sizes: 30A–38F
Prices: starts £10 for briefs; £20 for bras
Enquiries: 01525 851122

Hanro

Swiss high-quality underwear, with emphasis on fabrics (they use cashmere and silk among others). Highly technical fabrics used for bras, knickers, vests and bodies. Always black, white and cream, plus others according to fashion.

Sizes: knickers XS–L; bras 32A–38D
(not in every style)
Prices: from £14 for briefs; from £30 for
bras
Enquiries: 0171 245 6231

Harrods
Brands include Aubade, August Silk,
Berlei, Bonsoir, Calvin Klein, Christian
Dior, Daniel Hanson, Warners,
Chantelle, Triumph, Hanro, La Perla,
Sloggi, Lejaby, Rigby and Peller, Dolce
and Gabbana, Marilyn Monroe,
Princesse Tam Tam, Egeria, Laurence
Tavernier, Fantasie, Gossard, Louis
Feraud, Saxon, Piklik, Valentino, Veil,
Daniel Hanson, Tuttabankem. Exclu-
sive UK stockist of Prada.
Sizes: 30AA–40HH
Prices: from £5.95 for knickers to
£2,000 for a cashmere robe
Enquiries: 0171 730 1234

Harvey Nichols
Ranges include Cherchez la Femme,
Collette Dinnigan, Dolce and Gabbana,
Donna Karan, Fifi Chachnil, La Perla,
Malizia, Marvel, Rigby and Peller.
Sizes: cup sizes A–G
Prices: £15–£275
Enquiries: 0171 235 5000

House of Fraser
Brands include Playtex, Triumph, Gos-
sard, Berlei, Warners, Charnos,
Chantelle, Loveable, Fantasie, Rigby
and Peller, Ballet, Sloggi, Malizia, La
Perla, Calvin Klein and other fashion
brands. Anita mastectomy swimwear
also available, as are Royce and Emma-
Jane nursing bras.
Sizes: 30AA–44H
Prices: briefs £9–£15; bras around £20,
can range up to £150
Enquiries: 0171 963 2236

Jockey for Her
Thermal and microfibre T-shirts, leg-
gings, briefs, shorts and vests in navy,
red or white.
Sizes: 10–16
Prices: from £9
Enquiries: 0191 491 0088

John Lewis
Many brands, including Gossard,
Charnos, Warners, Triumph, Sloggi,
Playtex, La Perla, Ballet and Berlei.
Backless, strapless, multi-way, bridal
basques, seamless, underwired, shock
absorbers, nursing, maternity, 'Ultra-
bras', 'Wonderbras' and silicon breast
enhancers all available. Bras can be sent
away to have mastectomy pockets fitted
for a small charge.
Sizes: 32AA–44H
Prices: from £6.95
Enquiries: 0171 629 7711

John Smedley
Simple, sporty bra tops and knickers in
sea-island cotton or 100 per cent wool.
Sizes: S, M and L
Prices: start at £13 for cotton knickers
Enquiries: 0171 580 5075

Kenzo Lingerie
Pretty and exquisite bras and briefs;
modern and feminine but no lace.
Sizes: 32A–38C
Prices: £35–£65 for bras
Enquiries: 0171 584 2427

Knickerbox
Cotton, satin and lace fashionable, sim-
ple underwear.
Sizes: 32A–38C and 8–16
Prices: briefs from £4; bras from £14
Enquiries: 0171 284 1744

La Perla
World's leading underwear brand, with
a wide choice, including lacy, plain and
embroidered; mail order available.
Sizes: 32B–38D (not in every style)
Prices: from £50 for knickers; from £80
for bras
Enquiries: 0171 436 5864; mail order
0171 491 0503

La Perla Studio
Modern, plain styling in tulle and cot-
ton; good value for money.
Sizes: 32B–38D, but not across all styles
Prices: from £50 for bra; from £25 for
briefs
Enquiries: 0171 436 5864

La Senza
Bras, briefs and cami-sets available in latest colours and fabrics.
Sizes: 32A–40E
Prices: bra and briefs sets from around £20
Enquiries: 0171 831 1000

Malizia by La Perla
Diffusion line from La Perla, aimed at younger market.
Sizes: 32B–38D, but not across all styles
Prices: bras from £50; briefs from £20
Enquiries: 0171 436 5864

Margaret Ann
Selection of finest silks and satins available in standard sizes and a bespoke service available mail order. Can also supply traditional thermal underwear. Mastectomy, nursing, elderly, size 30+ and large-busted all very well catered for. Appointments necessary. Holder of a 'Dear Annie' Gold Star for excellence [see 'Gold Stars' chapter].
Sizes: 6–30, up to J cup; bras 54" backs and bespoke up to any size
Prices: right across the board
Enquiries: 01985 840520

Marks and Spencer
The nation's favourite place to buy underwear: lacy, sporty, cotton, silk, thermal, secret support, etc., etc., etc.
Sizes: knickers 8–22; bras 32AA–42DD and 40F (not in every style)
Prices: knickers from £3; bras from £10
Enquiries: 0171 935 4422

Marvel (La Perla)
Extravagant colours and styling, the most raunchy of the La Perla ranges.
Sizes: 32–38 in mostly B cups, sometimes Cs and Ds in certain styles
Prices: from £65 for bras; from £35 for briefs
Enquiries: 0171 436 5864

Medimac
Mastectomy specialists stocking their own brand, 'Nearly Me', and others. Appointments are necessary for free fitting but there is also a mail-order catalogue. Prosthesis available.

Sizes: 32AA–46DD
Prices: from £13.99
Enquiries: 01273 441436

Playtex
A bra for everyone, including the 'Wonderbra', 'Fits Beautifully' for the larger lady, 'Cherish' (tummy-control pants), 'Affinity' (everyday underwired bras), 'Cross Your Heart', 'Superlook Secrets' (control panel briefs), 'Wonderbra Bliss' (more subtle sister to the 'Wonderbra': i.e., everyday cleavage) and '18 Hours' (girdles and corselets for larger ladies).
Sizes: 32AA–46E
Prices: from £6
Enquiries: 0500 362430

Rigby and Peller
Holders of the Royal Warrant, making ornate expensive bras, briefs and bodies. All staff give personal fitting advice; there is also a made-to-measure service at the actual R&P shops. A large selection of mastectomy bras, including the R&P own label; pockets can be sewn in for £25 per pocket.
Sizes: 30–40, A–G (not in every style)
Prices: £19–£98
Enquiries: 01536 760282

Selfridges
Brands stocked include La Perla, Triumph, Calvin Klein, Gossard, Warners, Rigby and Peller, Fantasie, Emporio Armani, Dolce and Gabbana, Playtex, Charnos, Lejaby, Chantelle. Mastectomy service and advice available.
Sizes: 30AA–48HH (not right across the range)
Prices: bras £20–£160; briefs £8–£80; bodies £25–£250
Enquiries: 0171 629 1234

Shapely Figures from Ambrose Wilson
Mail-order lingerie, specializing in larger sizes
Sizes: 34–54, A–H
Prices: from £9.99 for a pack of two bras
Enquiries: 0800 262717 (quoting AWL2499)

Sloggi
Soft, sporty underwear in high-quality

cotton and Lycra. All bras have seamless cups. Ranges include '100' (white waistband with blue motif), '200' (wider waistband), '300' (very simple and especially soft fabrics with double gussets), '400' (the newest younger range, predominantly white, with some black and seasonal colours).
Sizes: bras 30AA–38D/40C; briefs 10–30 (44")
Prices: start at £4.50
Enquiries: 01793 720232

Sock Shop
Core ranges of classic and cosmetic (sheer moulded) ranges, as well as a cotton-jersey range and luxurious fashion ranges (plunge bras, etc.).
Sizes: 34A–36C (selected lines to D cup)
Prices: £6.99 (core range), from £19.99 (summer range) and from £29.99 (Christmas range)
Enquiries: 01524 271071; also mail order branch on 0171 329 3791

Taillissime
Mail-order bras, briefs and all-in-ones for larger sizes.
Sizes: 14–30, some in C–E cup
Prices: from £19.99 for a bra; from £9.99 for briefs
Enquiries: 0500 777777

Triumph
Strapless, minimizing, bridal, maternity and sports bras available in black, white, skin tones and fashion colours; plunge, seamless and padded cups also available. Some styles available mail order.
Sizes: 30AA–46H (not full size range in all styles); emphasis on fuller cup fittings
Prices: from £19
Enquiries: 01793 720232

Valentino Intimo
A luxurious range which reflects the mainline collection. Sheers and black, white and seasonal colours available.
Sizes: 32A–36D
Prices: from £17 for briefs; from £47 for a bra
Enquiries: 0115 9795796

Valisere
Traditional French lacy lingerie; lots of G-strings, camisoles, bras and briefs, with emphasis on colours.
Sizes: 32A–40DD
Prices: briefs from £25; bras from £40
Enquiries: 01793 720232

Warners
Ranges include 'Friday Bra' (very plain), 'Lace Perfection' (more glamorous), 'Body Beautiful' (emphasis on good fit), 'Supernaturals' (innovative fabrics), 'Leandra' (hand-painted range), 'Body Beware' (classical range), 'Pure Passion' (clean range), 'Simply Sensational' (modern clean range), 'Young Attitude' (fun range), 'Naked Truth' (totally sheer range), 'Velvet Beware' (high fashion), 'Not So Innocent Nudes' (opaque range), 'Sheer Luxury' (highly embroidered), 'Body Classics' (simple, light embroidery), 'Feronia' (classical bras) and 'Marilyn Monroe'.
Sizes: 32A–38FF (most ranges 32A–38E)
Prices: £9 thong; £38 bra
Enquiries: 0115 979 5796

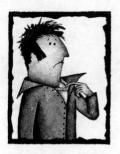

menswear

Anything and everything to help you if you are a man: big sizes, small sizes, unusual sizes, hiring, traditional . . .

Alfred Dunhill
48 Jermyn Street, London SW1Y 6LX
T 0171 290 8600
Traditional luxury menswear and
accessories, including shirts, suits, cufflinks, jewellery and fragrance. Masses
of services, including a complimentary
tie-loaning service (for businessmen's
lunches), personal shopping, a humidor
room, complimentary jewellery polishing, tailoring services, a steaming service, a Reuters screen and even a ladies'
section.

Angels Fancy Dress
119 Shaftesbury Avenue,
London WC2 8AE
T 0171 836 5678
Fancy-dress and costume hire, including
the actual costumes worn in many films
and TV productions. All periods are
covered, wigs and accessories available
too, and a wedding collection of period
costumes to hire. Must ring up and give
measurements, stating what is required.
A full costume costs from £70.50 for one
week plus £100 returnable deposit
required on every costume.

Atlas Man's Shop
197 Cricklewood Broadway,
London NW2 3HS
T 0181 450 6556
Atlas – who provide a very helpful and
friendly service – specialize in 'King'
sizes for men who can't find clothing to
fit them. Mainly casual wear, as well as
underwear, swimwear, dressing gowns
and some sportswear. Sizes often go up
to XXXXXXXXL, collar sizes go up to

23", trousers and jeans up to 60" waist,
and shirts up to 70" chest. Suit jackets
go up to 62" chest with XL bodies and
sleeves. Prices are around £21.99 for
shirts and from £150 for suits. Atlas also
do extra-tall trousers with up to 38"
inside leg (up to 44" waist) for £49.99.

Austin Reed
T 0800 585479 for enquiries;
branches nationwide
Three collections, including 'Austin
Reed', which is the classic suit label,
'AR', which is contemporary suiting,
and 'Reed', a casual younger range of
less structured separates. Also 'Sport
Reed' leisurewear, including swimwear.
Off-the-peg suits start at £250. Made-to-
measure service for suits starts at £300
and takes three–six weeks.

Ben Sherman
T 0800 592549 for stockists and enquiries
Ben Sherman has been selling its classic
button-down woven checked shirts
since 1963. There are three fits of the
shirts: classic, slim fit and easy fit. They
also stock trousers, knitwear, branded
leather goods (belts, jackets, etc.) and
footwear. Sizes S–XXL and boys' sizes
available too. Prices from £30.

Bertie Wooster
659 Fulham Road, London SW6 5PY
T 0171 371 0528
284 Fulham Road, London SW10 9BW
T 0171 352 5662
69 Moorgate, London EC2R 6BH
T 0171 638 9550
BW sell made-to-measure, traditionally
tailored menswear. Prices start at £350

for a two-piece suit and it takes about six weeks. Their shop on the Fulham Road also provides a hiring service for formal wear (prices start at £60 to hire a dinner jacket) and it also sells good-quality second-hand men's clothes: e.g., a Savile Row suit would cost about £110.

Boden
T 0181 453 1535 for mail order
Outdoor clothing, suiting sold as sepa-rates and lots of khaki casual wear. For-mal trousers are £60–£85, and jackets start at £115. Jackets are sized 38"–46" chest, trousers 30"–44" waist and come unfinished, can be finished to specifica-tions. For £4 a swatch book can be ordered for the suiting fabrics.

Burberry
165 Regent Street, London W1R 8PH
T 0171 734 5929 for stockists and enquiries
Complete menswear range, including suits, classic Crombie shirts, casual shirts, yachting wear, shoes and acces-sories. Their famous raincoat starts at £400. Sizing S–XL, trousers 30"–42" waist, all suit trousers come unfinished, in-store alterations. Mail-order cata-logue includes a selection of classics (0171 930 7803).

Burro
19a Floral Street, London WC2E 9DS
T 0171 240 5120
Designer and directional clothing for younger men. Stock labels such as G Lang and Klurk, and others according to season. Own range of quirky under-wear and swimwear in fabrics such as gingham. Prices start at £75 for a shirt and trousers from £85. Sample sales twice a year.

C&A
T 0171 629 1244 for customer services; branches nationwide
Very realistically priced clothes for all occasions, including sports (especially ski wear), casual, suiting, underwear, hats and shoes. All ages catered for. Sizes in some styles can go up to 52" chest, 50" waist and 21" collar. 550 stores throughout Europe.

Ermenegildo Zegna
37 New Bond Street, London W1Y 9HB
42 Shelton Street, London WC2H 9H
T 0171 493 4471 for enquiries and regional stockists
Textile manufacturer and leading Italian designer menswear label selling suiting and casual wear. Prices start at £99 for a shirt; soft suits are from £449. There is also a made-to-measure service offered.

Etro
14 Old Bond Street, London W1X 3DB
T 0171 495 5767 for stockists and enquiries
Traditional Italian menswear with a quirky twist. Lots of luxurious cashmere scarves, leather belts and gloves, as well as suiting and casual wear. Prices start at £49 for a belt and range to £552 upwards for a two-piece suit.

Favourbrook
T 0171 491 2337 for stockist/ mail-order enquiries
Favourbrook make frock coats, Nehru-collar jackets, two-piece suits, waistcoats and accessories in an endless selection of beautiful fabrics. Prices start at £70 for a shirt, £120 for a waistcoat and £380 for a jacket. There is also a made-to-order service. Customers can choose from over 2,500 fabrics to have a piece made according to a style which already exists.

Fenwick
New Bond Street, London W1A 3BS
T 0171 629 9161
Labels stocked include Kenzo, Joseph, Nicole Farhi, Paul Smith, John Smedley, 120% Linen, Duchamp, Etro and Panama (including underwear from Calvin Klein and Paul Smith). Trousers are generally sizes 30"–36" waist and 38"–44" chest for suits and jackets. Alter-ations on all unfinished trousers are free, and there is also an alteration service on

sleeves, waists, etc. Personal shopping and a mail order service are available.

French Connection
T 0171 399 7200 for enquiries; branches nationwide

FC sells casual wear, knitwear and formal wear, as well as shoes, underwear and various accessories. There is always a range of basics for every season, including jeans, sweaters and various moleskin pieces. Prices start at around £20 for a T-shirt and go up to £500 for a leather jacket. There are selected menswear items in 'FCUK Buy Mail' (0870 606 3285) and the 'Bathroom Collection' of smellies is unisex.

Greenfibres
Westbourne House, Plymouth Road, Totnes TQ9 5NB
T 01803 8680001
F 01803 868002

Mail-order company whose garments are produced from environmentally responsible fabrics and manufactured in socially responsible conditions using organic cotton, organic linen and hemp. Prices are £96 for hemp jeans, Oxford shirts from £48, socks from £6.50. Sizes S–XL, trousers 30"–38" waist and socks up to size 11. Lines are open 10 a.m.–9 p.m., Mon–Fri, and 12 a.m.–4 p.m., Sat.

Hackett
137 Sloane Street, London SW1X 9AY
T 0171 730 3331; branches in London only

Formal wear, casual wear and sportswear. Suiting can be made to order (prices start at £395) or bespoke (prices start at £800). Chinos cost from £49 and moleskin trousers cost from £69. Jacket sizes start at 36" chest short length and go up to 48" long length. All trousers are unfinished and can go up to length 38". A free mail-order catalogue is available from the above telephone number.

Harrods
Knightsbridge, London SW1X 7XL
T 0171 730 1234

Harrods men's departments include Way In (emphasis on casual and club-wear, aimed at fifteen–twenty-four-year-olds), Men's Casuals (smart and casual wear, including brands such as Hugo Boss, Marlboro Classics, Dockers, Gant USA, Armani Jeans), Manshop (shoes, suits, knits, hats, walking sticks, overcoats, umbrellas, wasicoats, bow ties and dressing gowns), and Men's Designer Collections (including Helmut Lang, Clements Ribeiro, John Rocha, PS, Jil Sander and Gucci boutiques). Way In prices start at £54.95 (sizes: waists 28"–38", inside leg 28"–36"), T-shirts and knitwear from £39.95 (sizes S–XXL). Men's Casuals jeans from £69. Manshop shirts from £42.95 (collar sizes 14½"–18"; 20" available in some styles and larger sizes can be ordered); ties £11.95–£299. Men's Designer Collections suits from £379 (sizes: 38"–46").

Henry Poole and Co.
15 Savile Row, London W1X 1AE
T 0171 734 5985; F: 0171 287 2161

The oldest bespoke tailor in London; former clients include Charles Dickens and Queen Victoria. Henry Poole has Royal Patronage and will travel worldwide to clients. A three-piece suit takes about a month, starting price £1,565 + VAT. Two-piece suits are from £1465 + VAT; blazers from £1,035 + VAT; sports jackets from £985 + VAT; and trousers from £495 + VAT.

Higginbotham Traditional Nightwear
T 01379 668833 for mail order and enquiries

Higginbotham's mail-order nightwear is all made from 100 per cent two-fold cotton poplin. Traditional nightshirts, pyjamas, kimonos and dressing gowns all made to traditional designs (e.g., self-fabric drawstrings and spare buttons). Available in a choice of traditional stripes in four colourways. Sizing is generous: S–XL (if in doubt, customers should go down a size rather than up), chest sizes up to 55". Prices from £45 (nightshirts) to £75 (dressing gowns), p&p is £3. Brochure available on request.

High and Mighty
T 0800 521542 for enquiries;
twenty-three shops nationwide
Retail and mail-order formal and casual
wear for tall and large men. High and
Mighty stock their own label and others.
Clothes for 'King Size' men are 44"–60"
chest, 40"–60" waist and 17"–21" collars. 'Tall' clothes are 40"–52" chest,
32"–48" waist, with inside leg up to 40".
There is also a larger-size shoe range
covering sizes 11–15, as well as many
other accessories: belts, etc. Prices start
at £14.95 for shirts and go up to £199 for
suits. Call 0845 601 0212 for a free catalogue.

Hugo Boss
T 0171 589 5522 for enquiries;
stockists nationwide
Two collections available. BOSS Hugo
Boss is the more traditional core brand,
with suiting, casual wear and separates.
Suits are from £379. HUGO Hugo Boss
is more avante-garde, aimed at the
younger market. Prices for shirts start at
£69, available from the Hugo Boss shops
and department stores. Hugo Boss
recently introduced a Golf range.

Index Extra
T 0345 979797 for mail order
In this mail-order catalogue men can
order shirts with extra-long sleeves or
trousers with extra-short leg lengths.
Some jackets are sized up to 52" chest,
some shirts go up to 19" collar and some
trousers up to 50" waist.

John Lewis
T 0171 629 7711 for enquiries;
branches nationwide
A full range of menswear is available,
including casual, formal, sports, underwear and nightwear. Many leading
brands stocked, as well as JL own brand,
Jonelle. There is a made-to-measure service available on suiting and an alterations service which is chargeable. There
is a massive selection of accessories,
from driving gloves at £19 (sizes 8–12)
and cufflinks (from £3.95 to £300 for an

antique pair) to Panama hats and Tril-
bys. Bed and bath towelling robes can
be made to order.

John Richmond
2 Newburgh Street, London W1V 1LH
T 0171 978 5278 for stockist enquiries
Mainline collection includes suiting and
tailoring as well as some knitwear. Prices
start at £550 for suiting. There is also a
John Richmond Denim collection, which
includes denims, combats and T-shirts.
Jeans start at £80. Trousers are available
to 34" length on unfinished hems. Shoes
available in both collections.

John Smedley
T 0171 734 1519 for enquiries;
stockists nationwide
Sea-island cotton jumpers available in
summer and merino wool jumpers in
winter. Sizes XS–XL in selected styles,
most sized S–XL. Prices from £60.

Johnsons
293 Portobello Road, W10
T 0181 964 3332
406 King's Road, London SW10 0LJ
T 0171 351 3268
Opening soon on Portobello Road; Kensington Market branch to be closed soon
Updated 1950s-, 1960s- and 1970s-influ-
enced clothing with a rock 'n' roll feel.
Jackets, jeans, frock coats, fake-fur
coats, highly coloured 1960s-style jackets, as well as lots of Vegas-style accessories: e.g., old LED watches, cufflinks,
Elvis sunglasses. Lots of the La Rocka –
Johnsons own label (including Donnie
Brasco-style Hawaiian shirts and col-
lege-style 1950s and 1960s shirts).

Jones
13–15 Floral Street, London WC2E 9DH
T 0171 240 8312
Two shops on Floral Street selling men's
designer wear, one geared more towards
designer mainlines (McQueen, Issey
Miyake, Helmut Lang, Costume
Homme, etc.) and the other carrying
more casual 'street' labels and a denims
(Final Homme, Marharishi, Evisu, etc.)
They do cater for a lot of very small and

trendy men, apparently, and sizes are XS–L. Prices start at £20 for a T-shirt in the casual wear. Mail order by cheque is possible if seen in the press. Alterations are free except on sale items.

Joseph
74 Sloane Avenue, London SW3 3DZ
T 0171 591 0808
Including the Joseph own label of suiting, separates, ties and 'Essentials'. Joseph also stocks top men's designers such as Gucci, luxury luggage from Valextra, Manolo Blahnik shoes and Robert Tateossian accessories. Sizes are S–XL; in-store alterations.

Land's End Direct Merchants
Pillings Road, Oakham,
Rutland LE15 6NY
T 0800 220106 for mail order and
enquiries
Land's End mail-order catalogue includes American-style trousers, casual shirts, formal shirts, sports jackets, outerwear, ties and accessories. As well as 'Men's Regular' sizes, Land's End offers 'Men's Tall' (proportionately longer in the torso and sleeves), 'Men's Big', and 'Men's Big and Tall' on selected items. Lines are open twenty-four hours a day, seven days a week, and all sales staff can advise on sizing and garment care. All items are 'Guaranteed Period', which means they can be returned at any time for a full refund or exchange.

Margaret Howell
29 Beauchamp Place, London SW3 1NJ
T 0171 584 2462 for stockist enquiries
Traditional shirts, suits and ties, but quite unstructured in styling. Lots of linens used in summer. Sizing is quite generous, as trousers are often loose. Lovely duffel coats from £325.

Marks and Spencer
T 0171 935 4422 for enquiries;
branches nationwide
M&S sell suits, jackets, trousers, shirts, accessories, underwear, nightwear and footwear for men. Jackets are sized 38"–48" chest (short and long length)

and 50" is available to order; shirt collars are sized 14½"–17½" and some shirts are available with an 18" collar. A direct catalogue is being trialled in SE England and Scotland which will include a selection of menswear. Currently made-to-measure suits are available only in the Finsbury Pavement branch.

Morgan Homme
T 0171 383 2888 for enquiries; available
only in concessions at the moment
French high street clothing aimed at twenty-five–fortyish men. Lots of pinstripe suiting, as well as casual suiting, denims, combats and T-shirts. Trousers are sized M–XXL, shirts S–XL.

Next
T 0116 284 9424 for stockist enquiries;
0345 100500 for mail order
All menswear covered in the shops and in the twice-yearly catalogues. Jackets are sized 36"–48" chest in short, regular and long dimensions (depends on chest sizing); formal trousers are sized 28"–38" waist in short, regular and longer lengths, and 40" waists come in regular and longer lengths; shirt collars 14½"–18". Boys' sizes available up to thirteen years. Casual shirts start at £24.99 and a full suit starts at £150. Some stores offer a semi-bespoke service: fabrics and linings can be chosen from the fabric book; specifications such as more buttons or no trouser pleats can be stated. It takes four–five weeks and starts at £260.

Nicole Farhi
55–56 Long Acre, London WC2E 9JL
T 0171 240 5240
Relaxed but smart tailoring, very easy to wear, with fantastic knitwear. Suits can be bought as separates and all trousers come unfinished and can be tailored to the right length. Sizes are 28"–38" waist trousers, jackets 38"–46" and collars 14½"–17½". Prices start at £199 for trousers and £399 for jackets.

Nigel Curtiss
T 0171 935 1314 for enquiries

Tailoring and casual wear in technically advanced, unusual fabrics: e.g., stainless-steel velvet. Sizes XS–XL; trousers are unfinished. Prices £85–£260 for shirts, £90–£240 for trousers and £250–£400 for jackets.

Racing Green
T 0990 411111 for mail order
Mail-order men's casual and outdoor wear, including jeans, chinos and cords. Sizes S–XXL for shirts. Trousers are available waist 30"–40" in different leg lengths: short (30"), regular (32"), long (34") and extra long (36"). Prices are from around £29 for shirts and from £32 for jeans.

Ralph Lauren
143 New Bond Street, London W1Y 9FD
T 0171 491 4967
Purple label by Ralph Lauren only available at the above address. Semi-bespoke suits (i.e., finishing details such as arm lengths can be adjusted) start from £1,500. The Polo Ralph Lauren line is also available at the New Bond Street shop (and branches nationwide: phone above number for details). Suiting and shirts. Prices from £55 for shirts. Polo Sport Ralph Lauren is the sportswear line and there is also an underwear range. Finally, the Polo Jeans Co. Ralph Lauren is the denims, sports and casual line, available at stockists nationwide (enquiries for this range: 0171 647 6500).

Rokit
225 Camden High Street, London, NW1 0NS
T 0171 267 3046
23 Kensington Gardens, Brighton, East Sussex BN1 4AL
T 01273 672053
Vintage clothing of the highest quality from the 1930s to the 1980s. Sourced mostly from North America, jeans start from £10. Many accessories such as shoes, belts and hats also available.

Schmidt Natural Clothing
21 Post Horn Close, Forest Row, East Sussex RH18 5DE
T 01342 822169 for mail order
Mail-order company selling natural clothing made from organic cotton, cotton with silk and silk with wool. For men there is mostly underwear, socks, slippers and nightwear. Sizes S–XL; socks and slippers up to size 14. Prices start at £5.90 for socks and £38.50 for pyjamas. Catalogues are free on the above number; lines open 9 a.m.–10 p.m., Mon–Sat.

Selfridges
Oxford Street, London W1
T 0171 629 1234
The menswear in this department store is divided up into three sections: formal wear (suiting from Armani, Ozwald Boateng, Gieves and Hawkes, as well as Gordon Selfridge – their own brand), casual collections (including Nautica, Ralph Lauren, Calvin Klein, Tommy Hilfiger) and designer wear (Helmut Lang, Dolce and Gabbana, etc.). Prices right across the board. There is also a Menswear Hair and Grooming Salon on the first floor and men's personal shopping on the second floor (call 0171 318 3223 for details).

Sports Locker
17 Floral Street, London WC2E 9DS
T 0171 240 4929
Men's underwear and sportswear, including swimwear. Labels stocked include Calvin Klein, Ralph Lauren, Russell Athletic. Tracksuits but no trainers. Sizes S, M and L. A mail-order catalogue is available; call for catalogue/further details.

The Natural Collection
T 01225 442288 for mail order
Mail-order company offering environmentally friendly clothing all made from organic cotton. Mostly leisurewear, including T-shirts, sweatshirts, joggers, briefs and bathrobes. Sweatshirts sized S–XL (34/36"–40/42") and joggers sized S–XL. Lines are open 9 a.m.–6 p.m., Mon–Fri, will deliver anywhere in the UK and catalogues are free.

The 1920s–1970s Crazy Clothes Connection
134 Lancaster Road, London W11 1QU
T 0171 221 3989

The CCC has hundreds of shirts, suits, overcoats, boots and all sorts of accessories from the 1920s to the 1970s available to hire or buy. The older stuff is mainly to hire only (deposit of £150 required). A full outfit starts at £50 to hire. Prices (to buy) start at £5 only and vary wildly. Open 1 p.m.–7 p.m., Mon, and 11 a.m.–7 p.m., Tues, Wed, Fri, Sat.

T. M. Lewin
T 0171 930 4291 for enquiries;
0800 376 1664 for mail order.
Four stores in London

Since 1898 T. M. Lewin have been offering mainly shirts. Dressing gowns, ties, boxer shorts, leather goods (wallets, etc.) and accessories such as cufflinks also sold. Casual shirts (i.e., corduroy) start at £39.50, and the formal shirts are priced £49.50—£65. Shirts are collar-size 14½"–18". T. M. Lewin has also collaborated with John Smedley to do some polo shirts (Smedley sea-island cotton used): long-sleeve are £69.50 and short-sleeve are £59.50. Casual shirts are sized S–XL. At the time of going to press, T. M. Lewin were looking into doing a bespoke service – call them for further details.

Tom Gilbey
2 New Burlington Place, Savile Row, London W1X 1FB
T 0171 734 4877; F 0171 434 2533

Fantasic groom service equal to that normally given to a bride; traditional and more contemporary tastes catered for. In addition to a hire service (individual garments from £55 for waistcoats), there is an off-the-peg service, which starts from £395, and a bespoke service from £1,250. Gilbey's waistcoat gallery has been established for about ten years: ready-to-wear from £130 and made-to-measure from £195; hand-painted or embroidered waistcoats are from 325. Also specializes in lightweight fabrics for overseas weddings.

Index

notes

notes

notes

notes

notes

notes

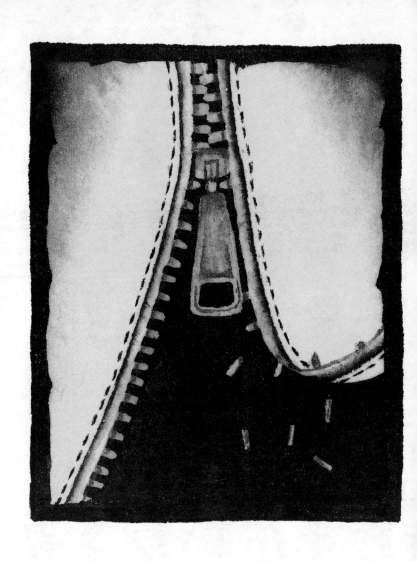